CARDIOLOGY RESEARCH AND CLINICAL DEVELOPMENTS

A HANDBOOK OF CARDIAC RESYNCHRONIZATION THERAPY WITH CASE STUDIES

CARDIOLOGY RESEARCH AND CLINICAL DEVELOPMENTS

Additional books in this series can be found on Nova's website under the Series tab.

Additional E-books in this series can be found on Nova's website under the E-book tab.

CARDIOLOGY RESEARCH AND CLINICAL DEVELOPMENTS

A HANDBOOK OF CARDIAC RESYNCHRONIZATION THERAPY WITH CASE STUDIES

RAJIV SANKARANARAYANAN
GRAEME KIRKWOOD
RAJAVARMA VISWESVARAIAH
AND
AMIR ZAIDI

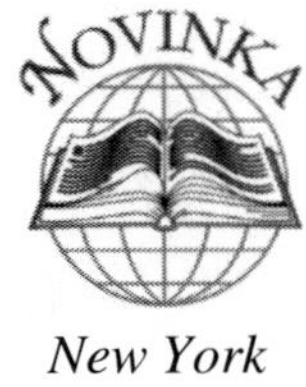

New York

Library of Congress Cataloging-in-Publication Data

Library of Congress Control Number: 2013931033

ISBN: 978-1-62618-029-1

Published by Nova Science Publishers, Inc. † New York

CONTENTS

PREFACE

Cardiac resynchronization therapy (CRT) is a relatively new treatment for heart failure which has come into prominence over the last decade as it produces significant improvements in morbidity and mortality over and above heart failure drug therapies. This is also a dynamic field with ever-improving implant techniques and an ever-increasing scope for patients who benefit from this therapy. Whilst the use of cardiac resynchronization is steadily increasing, studies and surveys worldwide have demonstrated that this life-saving therapy remains under-used possibly due to a lack of understanding of the indications and benefits of this therapy as well as a gap in knowledge regarding the management of patients who have CRT implants. This succinct yet thorough handbook contains eight chapters that will cover the historical developments of cardiac resynchronization therapy, the basics of heart failure, application of CRT in heart failure including implant techniques, management of complications, optimization techniques, as well as methods to minimize non-response of therapy by appropriate identification of patients who benefit from this treatment.

Chapter 1

HEART FAILURE

INTRODUCTION

Heart failure continues to impose a significant mortality and morbidity burden. Whilst heart failure can be caused by diverse conditions, these ultimately result in similar pathophysiological consequences of tissue hypoxia which initiates a vicious and ultimately detrimental neuro-hormonal compensatory cycle. Pharmacological therapies have consistently evolved, however these have not dented the mortality burden due to heart failure. It is essential to understand all these aspects of heart failure to fully appreciate the role of cardiac resynchronisation therapy in the multi-pronged management of heart failure.

EPIDEMIOLOGY

Chronic heart failure (CHF) is defined as a complex clinical syndrome due to any structural or functional cardiac abnormality that leads to the inability of the heart to effectively fill with or pump out blood and ultimately failure to supply enough oxygen for the metabolic demands of tissues [1, 2]. CHF has been recognised to have reached epidemic proportions in the 21st century [3]. With improved longevity leading to an ever increasing ageing population and the modern management of ischaemic heart disease (IHD) and CHF, also leading to improved survival, the prevalence of CHF continues to increase [4, 5]. The prevalence and incidence of CHF in the western world have been estimated to be 1- 2% and 5-10 per 1000 persons per year respectively [2, 6].

The prevalence of CHF in the USA is quoted to be over 5.8 million and the incidence is 550,000 [7]. About 2 million new cases of CHF are diagnosed worldwide and the world-wide prevalence of CHF is estimated to be 24 million [8, 9]. CHF also shows an increased incidence and prevalence amongst the elderly with the median age at initial presentation shown to be 76 years in one study [3, 6, 10].

In the Rotterdam study, the prevalence increased progressively with age (0.9% in subjects aged 55-64 years, 4% in those aged 65-74 years, 9.7% in age group 75-84 years and 17.4% in those aged over 85 years [3]. The incidence of CHF in this study also showed an age-dependant increase (from 2.5/1000 person years in subjects aged 55–64 years to 44/1000 person years in those 85 years or older) Other studies have also confirmed this increased propensity of CHF amongst the elderly [10, 11]. The Framingham Heart Study estimated that the a forty year old has a 1 in 5 lifetime risk of developing HF [12]. CHF has also been shown to be more common amongst men [3, 10]. Under the age of 65 years, there is a male predominance, above this age the sex distribution is more equitable [7].

Aetiology

The predominant cause of heart failure in the western world is IHD and has been identified to contribute to nearly half of the cases of CHF [13]. More than a third of patients have been shown to develop HF in the first eight years following a myocardial infarction [14].

Other aetiologies implicated include dilated cardiomyopathy, hypertension, valvular heart disease, diabetes, infections particularly viral, drugs (chemotherapeutic medication such as doxorubicin), toxins (alcohol, cocaine, amphetamine) and high-output metabolic states (pregnancy, beri-beri, thyrotoxicosis) [1].

Pathogenesis

The pathognomonic features of CHF are caused by a combination of tissue hypo-perfusion and the compensatory responses that attempt to counteract this.

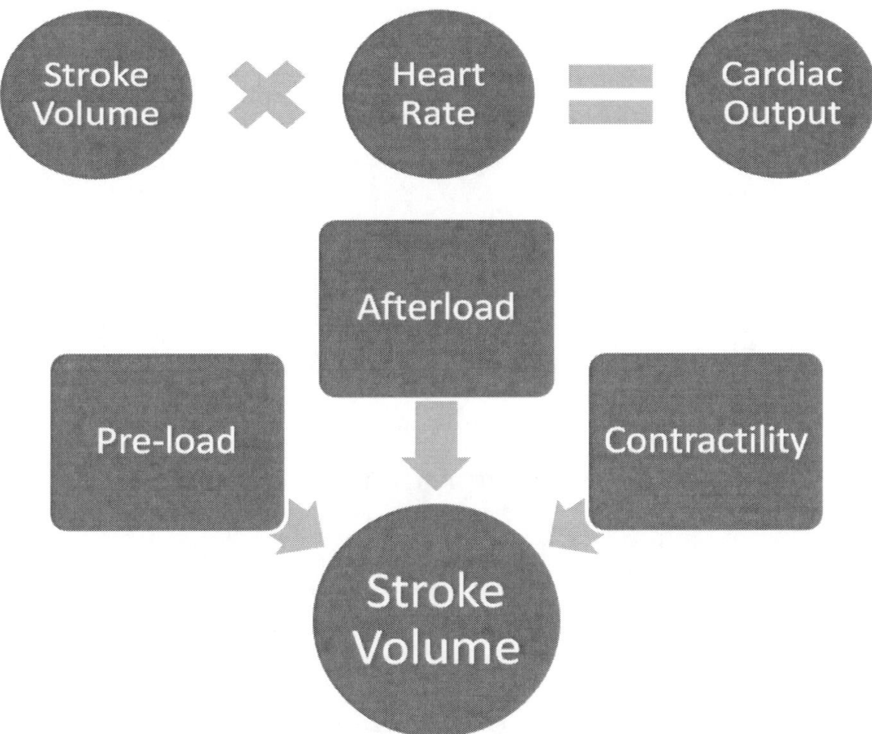

Figure 1. Factors influencing stroke volume.

One or more of the afore-mentioned aetiologies cause an initial cardiac insult leading to reduced cardiac output and global hypo-perfusion, ultimately triggering three major compensatory mechanisms (Frank-Starling mechanism, neuro-hormonal activation and ventricular remodelling).

Understanding normal cardiac physiology is crucial to unravel the pathogenesis of CHF. Normal cardiac output (CO) is between 4-8L/min and is determined by heart rate and stroke volume. Stroke volume (the amount of blood ejected every heart beat-about 1cc/kg), is in turn determined by pre-load (amount of blood that enters the left ventricle), contractility and after-load (the impedance to the left ventricular outflow). Pre-load is quantified in terms of left-ventricular end-diastolic volume, cardiac contractility is objectively described using ejection fraction (EF) and after-load is estimated using the mean arterial pressure. The inter-relationship between these factors is demonstrated in figure 1.

The Frank-Starling mechanism is a protective feature which operates generally during early stages of HF, whereby increased pre-load leads to increased left ventricular end-diastolic pressure and myocardial stretch, ultimately leading to increased CO [15, 16]. This mechanism is illustrated in figure 2 below.

The decrease in CO leads to a reduction in mean arterial pressure (MAP=CO X TPR).

As an early compensatory mechanism, neurohormonal activation increases TPR.

This is accomplished by catecholamine release (adrenaline and noradrenaline) through activation of the sympathetic nervous system.

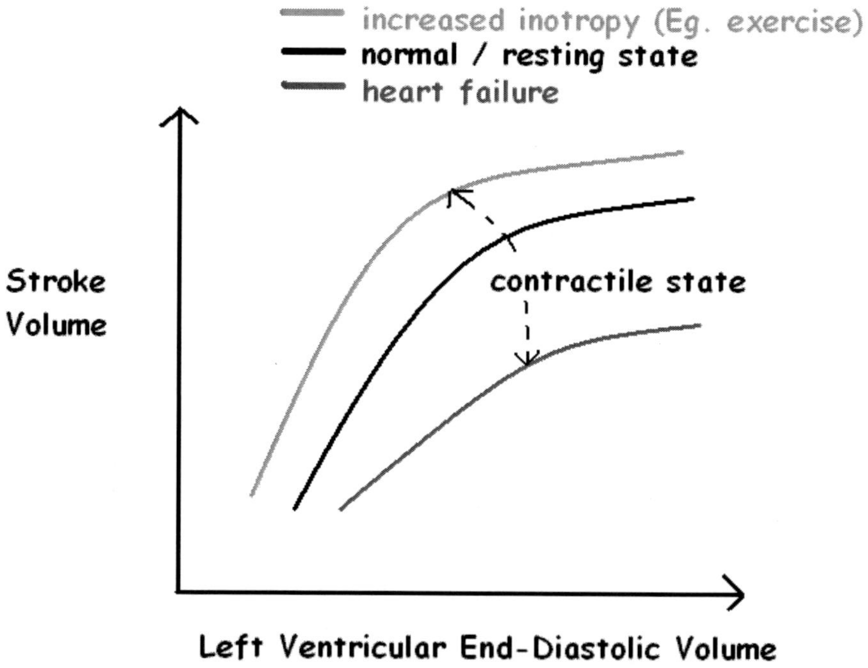

Figure 2. Frank-Starling Law illustrating the effects of LV end-diastolic volume on stroke volume and thus contractile state.

This and reduced renal blood flow stimulate the renal renin-angiotensin axis which leads to vasoconstriction, salt retention, vasopressin release and improved contractility [16, 17].

These effects are counter-acted by stretch-activated atrial and brain natriuretic peptides as well as vascular endothelial substances (nitric oxide, bradykinin and prostacyclin) which lead to vasodilation [18, 19]. CHF also leads to raised serum levels of cytokines such as TNFα, interferonα and interleukins which act as negative inotropes [20].

Prolonged neuro-hormonal activation is ultimately detrimental to the heart as it results in deleterious ventricular remodelling [16, 21]. This includes change in geometrical shape of the heart (becomes more spherical), increased ventricular mass and thickness and ultimately contractility [16, 17]. However, in the long run this compensation is also deleterious to contractility as it results in apoptosis and fibrosis.

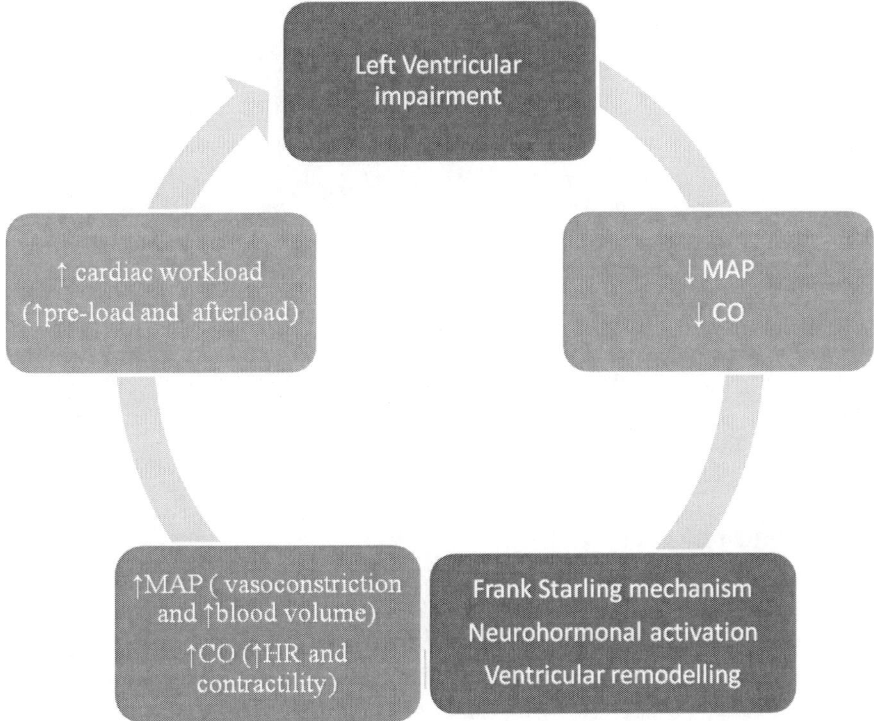

Figures 3 and 4. Diagrams illustrating the pathophysiological changes and compensatory mechanisms that constitute the vicious progressive cycle in heart failure.

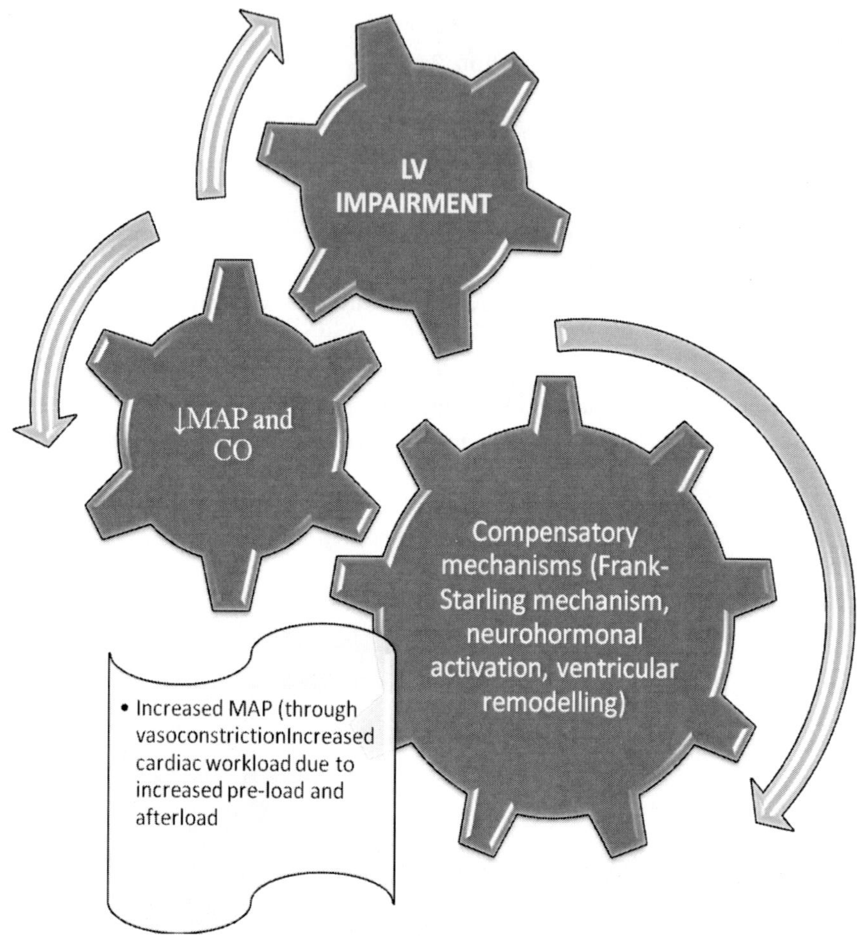

Figure 4. (Continued).

Assessment of Severity of CHF

The New York Heart Association (NYHA) functional classification of CHF grades CHF severity based on patient symptoms and level of physical activity (Table 1). In the United States about 70% CHF patients are estimated to be in NYHA Class I/II symptomatic status, 25% in Class III and the remaining 5% in Class IV [22]. The NYHA Classification is a simple and easy-to-interpret system; however it does possess some limitations.

Table 1. NYHA Classification of CHF symptoms (described in The Criteria Committee of the New York Heart Association Nomenclature and criteria for diagnosis of diseases of the heart and blood vessels. Boston: Little Brown, 1964)

NYHA CLASS	SYMPTOMS
I	No limitation of physical activity. Ordinary physical activity does not cause undue fatigue, palpitation, dyspnea, or angina
II	Slight limitation of physical activity. Ordinary physical activity results in fatigue, palpitation, dyspnea, or angina
III	Marked limitation of physical activity. Comfortable at rest, but less than ordinary physical activity results in fatigue, palpitation, dyspnea, or angina
IV	Unable to carry on any physical activity without discomfort. Symptoms are present at rest. With any physical activity, symptoms increase

These include poor correlation between symptom severity and ventricular function in addition to the fact that patients with mild symptoms can also experience adverse clinical events such as hospitalisation and death [23, 24]. It has been demonstrated however that mortality risk increases with worsening NYHA Class [25]. The contribution of heart failure itself to mortality increases with worsening NYHA Class (as a proportion of all deaths -12% in NYHA Class II patients, 26% in NYHA Class III and 56% in NYHA Class IV) [25]. In contrast, sudden cardiac deaths are more frequent amongst patients with milder NYHA Class (64% amongst NYHA Class II, 59% amongst Class III and 33% in Class IV patients). The ACC/AHA guidelines also describe four stages of CHF correlating presence of overt structural heart disease with symptoms and disease progression (Table 2) [1]. This system serves to illustrate the importance of treatment interventions prior to onset of symptoms or LV dysfunction, thus preventing progression of disease and also reducing mortality as well as morbidity due to the condition. This classification recommends a more individualized treatment strategy for patients in each stage as opposed to treatments which can be largely similar for patients despite varying NYHA Class. The Killip staging system grades the severity of CHF complicating acute MI [26].

Table 2. Drugs Recommended in the Management of Chronic Heart Failure with Reduced LVEF (At Least ⩽40%)

DRUG	ESC Guidelines Level of recommendation, Strength of Evidence	ACC/AHA	HFSA Level of recommendation, Strength of Evidence
ACE-inhibitor	IA	IA	IA
Beta-blocker	IA	IA	IA
Angiotensin Receptor Blockers	IA (If ACE-inhibitor intolerant) IA (If persisting symptoms dspite ACE-inhibitor and beta-blocker but intolerant of aldosterone antagonist)	IA (If ACE-inhibitor intolerant) II bB if persistent symptoms despite optimum therapy	A (if intolerance to ACE inhibitors) A (in addition to ACE inhibitor and beta-blocker if persistent or worsening symptoms)
Hydralazine and oral nitrate		IB(African Americans with moderate to severe symptoms despite optimum medical therapy) II aB(if persistent symptoms despite ACE inhibitor and beta-blocker) II bC if intolerant of both ACEinh and ARB	C(if intolerance to ACE and angiotensin receptor inhibitors) A (for African Americans)
Aldosterone Receptor Blockers	IA (if LVEF≤35% and persisting symptoms despite ACE/ARB and beta-blocker)	IB (patients with moderate to severe symptoms)	A (post-MI HF) A(severe HF with LVEF<35% and NYHA Class 4 or Class 3 with previous Class 4 symptoms despite combination therapy including ACE-inhibitors, beta-blocker,diuretic)

DRUG	ESC Guidelines Level of recommendation, Strength of Evidence	ACC/AHA	HFSA Level of recommendation, Strength of Evidence
Ivabradine	II aB (if LVEF≤35%,heart rate≥70 bpm, NYHA 2-4 symptoms despite OPT II bC – if LVEF≤35%,HR≥70 bpm and intolerant of beta-blocker		
Digoxin	II bB –if sinus rhythm, EF≤45% and intolerant of beta-blocker II bB- if EF≤45% and NYHA2-4 despite standard therapy	ΠaB (if current or previous symptoms of HF)	If symptomatic or signs of HF despite standard therapy and NYHA2-3 – B; NYHA 4 –C
Diuretic			A (patients with evidence of fluid overload)

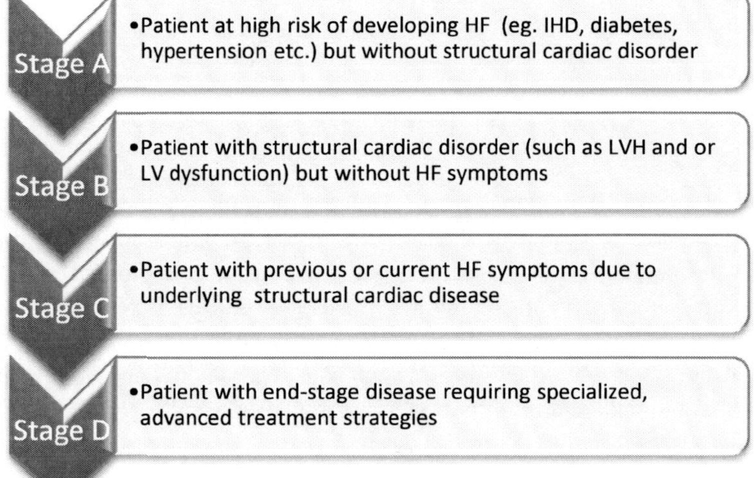

Figure 5. ACC/AHA Heart Failure Staging [1].

BURDEN

The diagnosis of CHF portends poor prognosis despite modern drug therapy [6], conferring a five year mortality risk varying from 41% (Rotterdam study) [3] to 65% (Framingham heart study) [12]. These mortality data are comparable to that conferred by some of the cancers [27, 28]. More than a third of all cardiovascular deaths in USA are attributable to CHF [7]. The short-term and medium-term mortality are significant as well due to a 10-20% one month mortality and 30% 1 year mortality [10]. More than three-quarters of patients require at least two hospital admissions each year and hospitalisation for CHF also predicts increased mortality risk (approximately 10% at 1 month, 22% at 1 year and about 42% at 5 years) [7, 29, 30, 31, 32, 33, 34]. The annual cost due to CHF is estimated to be between $10 to 38 billion [7, 33, 34]. Thus there is significant morbidity and mortality due to CHF despite advances in drug treatments. There is a contrast in the mode of death between various stages of CHF. Whilst arrhythmias and sudden cardiac death predominate in patients with mild to moderate heart failure (NYHA1-2), pump-failure deaths tend to occur more frequently amongst patients with severe and end-stage heart failure (NYHA 3-4) [6].

Whilst NYHA scoring system is a useful symptom severity score, the correlation to risk of hospitalisation is not robust and the mortality risk-prediction is not absolute either [23, 24, 35]. It has however been an important inclusion criterion in the landmark CRT trials.

OVERVIEW OF TREATMENT OF HF

The goals of CHF management include mortality reduction, symptom-relief, improvement in quality of life and exercise tolerance and prevention of hospitalisations due to CHF deterioration. Most large scale clinical trials have used mortality reduction and reduction in hospitalisations as primary outcome measures. Treatment of CHF includes life-style changes, risk-factor modification, treatment of aetiologies such as ischaemia, hypertension diabetes etc, pharmacological and non-pharmacological therapies.

Drug therapies include diuretics for pre-load reduction which helps relieve symptoms due to fluid overload and also improve exercise tolerance. Drugs with mortality benefit include ACE inhibitors/ARBs, beta-blockers and aldosterone antagonists. A combination of ACE-inhibitor, (or ARB if ACE-inhibitor intolerant) and beta-blocker is recommended (Class I, Level A) for all patients with HF and EF≤40% unless contra-indicated [1, 2]. ACE-inhibitors exert beneficial effects through interference with RAAS activation and thus retard long-term complications of this cascade such as cardiac remodelling [36, 37]. Evaluation of results from 30 randomised trials of a variety of ACE-inhibitors in approximately 7000 HF patients showed a statistically significant reduction in total mortality (odds ratio [OR], 0.77; 95% confidence interval [CI], 0.67 to 0.88; P < .001) and in the combined endpoint of mortality or hospitalization for congestive heart failure (OR, 0.65; 95% CI, 0.57 to 0.74; P < .001) [38]. Two of the early landmark trials which demonstrated the beneficial effects of ACE-inhibitors in HF were CONSENSUS (Co-operative North Scandinavian Enalapril Survival Study) and SOLVD-Treatment (Studies of Left Ventricular Dysfunction), both of which compared enalapril to placebo [39 40]. CONSENSUS showed significant mortality reduction in patients with severe heart CHF (Relative Risk Reduction 27% and Absolute Risk Reduction 14.6%) indicating a number needed to treat (NNT) of 7 (during an average of 6 months) [2, 39]. The corresponding figures in the SOLVD trial which randomised patients with mild to moderate HF were a mortality RRR of 16%, ARR 4.5% and NNT of 22 (average 41 months) [2, 41]. Beta-blockers inhibit the side-effects of compensatory catecholamine surges and their adverse consequences such as arrhythmias. A meta-analysis of 18 RCTs including over 3000 CHF patients showed that beta-blocker use leads to significant reduction in mortality (all-cause mortality reduction by 32%), combined risk of death or CHF hospitalisation reduced by 37%, and improvements in NYHA class as well as LVEF (increase by 29%) [42].

Key landmark trials which randomised approximately 9000 patients with mild to severely symptomatic CHF to beta-blocker or placebo (majority of who were also on ACE-inhibitors) included CIBIS II (Cardiac Insufficiency Bisoprolol Study II), MERIT-HF and COPERNICUS [25, 43, 44]. The inclusion criteria for these trials differed (CIBIS-II recruited patients with LVEF≤35% and NYHA III-IV symptoms, MERIT-HF recruited patients with LVEF≤40%, NYHA II-IV; COPERNICUS patients were much sicker with LVEF<25% and NYHA IV symptoms). There were significant reductions in total mortality in all three trials: CIBIS-II -HR = 0.77 [95% CI = 0.65–0.92] versus MERIT-HF -HR = 0.66 [0.54–0.81], HR = 0.66 [0.53–0.81], and COPERNICUS -HR = 0.65 [0.52–0.81], respectively. These included significant reductions in cardiovascular as well as sudden deaths. The RRR for mortality was about 34% in each of these trials and the RRR for HF hospitalisations was between 28% and 36% within a year on treatment. The ARR in mortality during a similar period in patients from both the CIBIS-II and MERIT-HF trials was 4.3% and NNT was 23 [2]. Results from the COPERNICUS trial showed an ARR of 7.1% and NNT of 14 [2]. These effects were in addition to those produced by ACE inhibitors as the majority of patients in these trials were also on ACE inhibitors.

Mineralocorticoid receptor antagonists such as spironolactone and eplerenone have been shown in the RALES (NYHA Class 3 symptoms and LVEF ≤35%) and EMPHASIS trials respectively (NYHA Class 2 symptoms and LVEF≤30%) to produce significant reductions in mortality as well as HF hospitalisations over and above those produced by ACE inhibitors and beta-blockers [45, 46]. Ivabradine (a sinus node I_f channel inhibitor) use in the SHIFT study of over 6500 patients with LVEF≤35%, NYHA Class 2-4 and heart rate≥70bpm, led to a significant reduction in the primary composite outcome of cardiovascular death or HF hospitalisation in addition to improvement in LV function and quality of life [47]. Digoxin has been shown to produce symptomatic benefit and prevent decompensation, without evidence of significant mortality benefit [2, 48].

Dyssynchrony and HF

In up to a third to half of patients with heart failure, there is an abnormality of inter-ventricular or intra-ventricular electrical conduction leading to inco-ordination of the sequence of regional or global left and right ventricular contraction [49, 50, 51]. The regional imbalances in systolic contraction lead to inefficient global LV pumping as parts of the LV wall are contracting against other parts which are relaxing [52, 53]. These patients usually present with a prolonged QRS duration of >120msec on ECG. Such findings have been associated with adverse cardiac haemodynamic consequences due to a combination of poor systolic function, impaired LV filling and also increased mitral regurgitation [53, 54, 55, 56], ultimately resulting in increased mortality [52, 57, 58]. Increasing inter and intra-ventricular conduction delay when in sinus rhythm can also potentiate lethal ventricular arrhythmias [59]. The Italian HF Registry analysis showed that patients with QRS duration>200 msec have a five times increased risk of death when compared to HF patients with narrow QRS [60].

Dyssonchronous heart failure has been shown to demonstrate marked heterogeneity in dysfunctional calcium handling as well as cellular electrophysiology varying in different walls of the LV. For instance in a canine tachypacing-induced HF model, the lateral wall is preferentially affected in down-regulation of calcium-handling proteins (30% reduction in SERCA, 80% reduction in phospholamban), 60% reduction in connexin 43 and also a two-fold increase in mitogen activated protein kinase [65]. The action potential duration has also been shown to be most prolonged in the late-activated lateral wall in dyssynchronous HF [66]. Similarly changes in the calcium transient are most marked in myocytes from the lateral wall (reduced calcium transient amplitude, slowed decay). Both anterior and lateral wall myocytes are characterised by down-regulation of potassium currents (inward rectifier- I_{K1}, delayed rectifier-I_K and transient outward potassium currents-I_{to}) [66].CRT has been shown to shorten action potential duration, restore rectifier-I_{K1}, delayed rectifier-I_K currents, increase calcium transient amplitude in lateral wall myocytes (but not anterior wall myocytes) and quicken the decay phase of the systolic calcium transient in both regions. In addition, CRT also improved the blunted contractile response to beta-adrenergic stimulation [67].

REFERENCES

[1] Hunt SA, Abraham WT, Chin MH, et al. 2009 Focused update incorporated into the ACC/AHA 2005 Guidelines for the Diagnosis and Management of Heart Failure in Adults A Report of the American College of Cardiology Foundation/American Heart Association Task Force on Practice Guidelines Developed in Collaboration With the International Society for Heart and Lung Transplantation. *J. Am. Coll. Cardiol.* 2009 Apr 14;53(15):e1-e90.

[2] McMurray JJ, Adamopoulos S, Anker SD, et al. ESC Guidelines for the diagnosis and treatment of acute and chronic heart failure 2012: The Task Force for the Diagnosis and Treatment of Acute and Chronic Heart Failure 2012 of the European Society of Cardiology. Developed in collaboration with the Heart Failure Association (HFA) of the ESC. *Eur. J. Heart Fail* 2012 Aug;14(8):803-69.

[3] Bleumink GS, Knetsch AM, Sturkenboom MC, et al. Quantifying the heart failure epidemic: prevalence, incidence rate, lifetime risk and prognosis of heart failure The Rotterdam Study. *Eur. Heart J.* 2004 Sep;25(18):1614-9.

[4] Senni M, Tribouilloy CM, Rodeheffer RJ, et al. Congestive heart failure in the community: trends in incidence and survival in a 10-year period. *Arch. Intern Med.* 1999 Jan 11;159(1):29-34.

[5] Gottdiener JS, Arnold AM, Aurigemma GP, et al. Predictors of congestive heart failure in the elderly: the Cardiovascular Health Study. *J. Am. Coll. Cardiol.* 2000 May;35(6):1628-37.

[6] Mosterd A, Hoes AW. Clinical epidemiology of heart failure. *Heart* 2007 Sep;93(9):1137-46.

[7] Roger VL, Go AS, Lloyd-Jones DM, et al. Heart disease and stroke statistics--2011 update: a report from the American Heart Association. *Circulation* 2011 Feb 1;123(4):e18-e209.

[8] McMurray JJ, Petrie MC, Murdoch DR, et al. Clinical epidemiology of heart failure: public and private health burden. *Eur. Heart J.* 1998 Dec;19 Suppl P:9-16.

[9] Cardiovascular Disease. World Health Organisation 2011 June 6 [cited 2011 Jun 6];Available from: URL: http://www.who.int/mediacentre/factsheets/fs317/en/index.html

[10] Cowie MR, Wood DA, Coats AJ, et al. Incidence and aetiology of heart failure; a population-based study. *Eur. Heart J.* 1999 Mar;20(6):421-8.

[11] Redfield MM, Jacobsen SJ, Burnett JC, Jr., et al. Burden of systolic and diastolic ventricular dysfunction in the community: appreciating the scope of the heart failure epidemic. *JAMA* 2003 Jan 8;289(2):194-202.

[12] Lloyd-Jones DM, Larson MG, Leip EP, et al. Lifetime risk for developing congestive heart failure: the Framingham Heart Study. *Circulation* 2002 Dec 10;106(24):3068-72.

[13] Fox KF, Cowie MR, Wood DA, et al. Coronary artery disease as the cause of incident heart failure in the population. *Eur. Heart J.* 2001 Feb;22(3):228-36.

[14] Hellermann JP, Goraya TY, Jacobsen SJ, et al. Incidence of heart failure after myocardial infarction: is it changing over time? *Am. J. Epidemiol.* 2003 Jun 15;157(12):1101-7.

[15] Westerhof N, O'Rourke MF. Haemodynamic basis for the development of left ventricular failure in systolic hypertension and for its logical therapy. *J. Hypertens* 1995 Sep;13(9):943-52.

[16] Kemp CD, Conte JV. The pathophysiology of heart failure. *Cardiovasc Pathol.* 2012 Sep;21(5):365-71.

[17] Young JB. Heart failure, ventricular remodelling and the renin-angiotensin system: insights from recently completed clinical trials. *Eur. Heart J.* 1993 Jul;14 Suppl C:14-7.

[18] Kim HN, Januzzi JL, Jr. Natriuretic peptide testing in heart failure. *Circulation* 2011 May 10;123(18):2015-9.
[19] Boulanger CM. Secondary endothelial dysfunction: hypertension and heart failure. *J. Mol. Cell Cardiol.* 1999 Jan;31(1):39-49.
[20] Chen D, ssad-Kottner C, Orrego C, et al. Cytokines and acute heart failure. *Crit. Care Med.* 2008 Jan;36(1 Suppl):S9-16.
[21] Curry CW, Nelson GS, Wyman BT, et al. Mechanical dyssynchrony in dilated cardiomyopathy with intraventricular conduction delay as depicted by 3D tagged magnetic resonance imaging. *Circulation* 2000 Jan 4;101(1):E2.
[22] What is heart failure? NHLBI 2011 [cited 2011 Jun 6];Available from: URL: http://www.nhlbi.nih.gov/health/dci/Diseases/Hf/HF_All.html
[23] McMurray JJ. Clinical practice. Systolic heart failure. *N. Engl. J. Med.* 2010 Jan 21;362(3):228-38.
[24] Chen J, Normand SL, Wang Y, et al. National and regional trends in heart failure hospitalization and mortality rates for Medicare beneficiaries, 1998-2008. *JAMA* 2011 Oct 19;306(15):1669-78.
[25] Effect of metoprolol CR/XL in chronic heart failure: Metoprolol CR/XL Randomised Intervention Trial in Congestive Heart Failure (MERIT-HF). *Lancet* 1999 Jun 12;353(9169):2001-7.
[26] Khot UN, Jia G, Moliterno DJ, et al. Prognostic importance of physical examination for heart failure in non-ST-elevation acute coronary syndromes: the enduring value of Killip classification. *JAMA* 2003 Oct 22;290(16):2174-81.
[27] Stewart S, MacIntyre K, Hole DJ, et al. More 'malignant' than cancer? Five-year survival following a first admission for heart failure. *Eur. J. Heart Fail* 2001 Jun;3(3):315-22.
[28] Askoxylakis V, Thieke C, Pleger ST, et al. Long-term survival of cancer patients compared to heart failure and stroke: a systematic review. *BMC Cancer* 2010;10:105.
[29] Fonarow GC, Adams KF, Jr., Abraham WT, et al. Risk stratification for in-hospital mortality in acutely decompensated heart failure: classification and regression tree analysis. *JAMA* 2005 Feb 2;293(5):572-80.
[30] Levy D, Kenchaiah S, Larson MG, et al. Long-term trends in the incidence of and survival with heart failure. *N. Engl. J. Med.* 2002 Oct 31;347(18):1397-402.

[31] Lucas C, Johnson W, Hamilton MA, et al. Freedom from congestion predicts good survival despite previous class IV symptoms of heart failure. *Am. Heart J.* 2000 Dec;140(6):840-7.

[32] MacIntyre K, Capewell S, Stewart S, et al. Evidence of improving prognosis in heart failure: trends in case fatality in 66 547 patients hospitalized between 1986 and 1995. *Circulation* 2000 Sep 5;102(10):1126-31.

[33] English MA, Mastrean MB. Congestive heart failure: public and private burden. *Crit. Care Nurs. Q* 1995 May;18(1):1-6.

[34] Havranek EP, Abraham WT. The health care economics of heart failure. *Heart Fail* 1998;14:10-8.

[35] Dunlay SM, Redfield MM, Weston SA, et al. Hospitalizations after heart failure diagnosis a community perspective. *J. Am. Coll. Cardiol.* 2009 Oct 27;54(18):1695-702.

[36] McDonald KM, Mock J, D'Aloia A, et al. Bradykinin antagonism inhibits the antigrowth effect of converting enzyme inhibition in the dog myocardium after discrete transmural myocardial necrosis. *Circulation* 1995 Apr 1;91(7):2043-8.

[37] Jessup M, Brozena S. Heart failure. *N. Engl. J. Med.* 2003 May 15;348(20):2007-18.

[38] Garg R, Yusuf S. Overview of randomized trials of angiotensin-converting enzyme inhibitors on mortality and morbidity in patients with heart failure. Collaborative Group on ACE Inhibitor Trials. *JAMA* 1995 May 10;273(18):1450-6.

[39] Swedberg K, Kjekshus J. Effects of enalapril on mortality in severe congestive heart failure: results of the Cooperative North Scandinavian Enalapril Survival Study (CONSENSUS). *Am. J. Cardiol.* 1988 Jul 11;62(2):60A-6A.

[40] Effect of enalapril on survival in patients with reduced left ventricular ejection fractions and congestive heart failure. The SOLVD Investigators. *N. Engl. J. Med.* 1991 Aug 1;325(5):293-302.

[41] Effect of enalapril on survival in patients with reduced left ventricular ejection fractions and congestive heart failure. The SOLVD Investigators. *N. Engl. J. Med.* 1991 Aug 1;325(5):293-302.

[42] Lechat P, Packer M, Chalon S, et al. Clinical effects of beta-adrenergic blockade in chronic heart failure: a meta-analysis of double-blind, placebo-controlled, randomized trials. *Circulation* 1998 Sep 22;98(12):1184-91.

[43] The Cardiac Insufficiency Bisoprolol Study II (CIBIS-II): a randomised trial. *Lancet* 1999 Jan 2;353(9146):9-13.

[44] Kindermann M, Bohm M. [Severe heart failure--effects of carvedilol therapy. The Copernicus Study]. *Internist (Berl)* 2002 Feb;43(2):284-6.

[45] Pitt B, Zannad F, Remme WJ, et al. The effect of spironolactone on morbidity and mortality in patients with severe heart failure. Randomized Aldactone Evaluation Study Investigators. *N. Engl. J. Med.* 1999 Sep 2;341(10):709-17.

[46] Zannad F, McMurray JJ, Krum H, et al. Eplerenone in patients with systolic heart failure and mild symptoms. *N. Engl. J. Med.* 2011 Jan 6;364(1):11-21.

[47] Ekman I, Chassany O, Komajda M, et al. Heart rate reduction with ivabradine and health related quality of life in patients with chronic heart failure: results from the SHIFT study. *Eur. Heart J.* 2011 Oct;32(19):2395-404.

[48] Hood WB, Jr., Dans AL, Guyatt GH, et al. Digitalis for treatment of congestive heart failure in patients in sinus rhythm: a systematic review and meta-analysis. *J. Card Fail* 2004 Apr;10(2):155-64.

[49] Aaronson KD, Schwartz JS, Chen TM, et al. Development and prospective validation of a clinical index to predict survival in ambulatory patients referred for cardiac transplant evaluation. *Circulation* 1997 Jun 17;95(12):2660-7.

[50] Farwell D, Patel NR, Hall A, et al. How many people with heart failure are appropriate for biventricular resynchronization? *Eur. Heart J.* 2000 Aug;21(15):1246-50.

[51] Wilensky RL, Yudelman P, Cohen AI, et al. Serial electrocardiographic changes in idiopathic dilated cardiomyopathy confirmed at necropsy. *Am. J. Cardiol.* 1988 Aug 1;62(4):276-83.

[52] Xiao HB, Roy C, Fujimoto S, et al. Natural history of abnormal conduction and its relation to prognosis in patients with dilated cardiomyopathy. *Int. J. Cardiol.* 1996 Feb;53(2):163-70.

[53] Littmann L, Symanski JD. Hemodynamic implications of left bundle branch block. *J. Electrocardiol.* 2000;33 Suppl:115-21.

[54] Xiao HB, Brecker SJ, Gibson DG. Effects of abnormal activation on the time course of the left ventricular pressure pulse in dilated cardiomyopathy. *Br. Heart J.* 1992 Oct;68(4):403-7.

[55] Saxon LA, Kerwin WF, Cahalan MK, et al. Acute effects of intraoperative multisite ventricular pacing on left ventricular function

and activation/contraction sequence in patients with depressed ventricular function. *J. Cardiovasc. Electrophysiol.* 1998 Jan;9(1):13-21.

[56] Kerwin WF, Botvinick EH, O'Connell JW, et al. Ventricular contraction abnormalities in dilated cardiomyopathy: effect of biventricular pacing to correct interventricular dyssynchrony. *J. Am. Coll. Cardiol.* 2000 Apr;35(5):1221-7.

[57] Shamim W, Francis DP, Yousufuddin M, et al. Intraventricular conduction delay: a prognostic marker in chronic heart failure. *Int. J. Cardiol.* 1999 Jul 31;70(2):171-8.

[58] Unverferth DV, Magorien RD, Moeschberger ML, et al. Factors influencing the one-year mortality of dilated cardiomyopathy. *Am. J. Cardiol.* 1984 Jul 1;54(1):147-52.

[59] Denniss AR, Richards DA, Cody DV, et al. Prognostic significance of ventricular tachycardia and fibrillation induced at programmed stimulation and delayed potentials detected on the signal-averaged electrocardiograms of survivors of acute myocardial infarction. *Circulation* 1986 Oct;74(4):731-45.

[60] Baldasseroni S, Opasich C, Gorini M, et al. Left bundle-branch block is associated with increased 1-year sudden and total mortality rate in 5517 outpatients with congestive heart failure: a report from the Italian network on congestive heart failure. *Am. Heart J.* 2002 Mar;143(3):398-405.

[61] Cahalin LP, Mathier MA, Semigran MJ, et al. The six-minute walk test predicts peak oxygen uptake and survival in patients with advanced heart failure. *Chest* 1996 Aug;110(2):325-32.

[62] Zugck C, Kruger C, Durr S, et al. Is the 6-minute walk test a reliable substitute for peak oxygen uptake in patients with dilated cardiomyopathy? *Eur. Heart J.* 2000 Apr;21(7):540-9.

[63] Weber KT, Kinasewitz GT, Janicki JS, et al. Oxygen utilization and ventilation during exercise in patients with chronic cardiac failure. *Circulation* 1982 Jun;65(6):1213-23.

[64] Mancini DM, Eisen H, Kussmaul W, et al. Value of peak exercise oxygen consumption for optimal timing of cardiac transplantation in ambulatory patients with heart failure. *Circulation* 1991 Mar;83(3):778-86.

[65] Spragg DD, Leclercq C, Loghmani M, et al. Regional alterations in protein expression in the dyssynchronous failing heart. *Circulation* 2003 Aug 26;108(8):929-32.

[66] Aiba T, Hesketh GG, Barth AS, et al. Electrophysiological consequences of dyssynchronous heart failure and its restoration by resynchronization therapy. *Circulation* 2009 Mar 10;119(9):1220-30.

[67] Chakir K, Daya SK, Aiba T, et al. Mechanisms of enhanced beta-adrenergic reserve from cardiac resynchronization therapy. *Circulation* 2009 Mar 10;119(9):1231-40.

Chapter 2

EVIDENCE-BASE FOR CRT

INTRODUCTION

Cardiac resynchronisation therapy (CRT) has now been firmly established as an important therapeutic option in the multi-pronged management strategy for chronic heart failure (CHF). The technique was first described about two decades ago and following small randomised studies showing the benefits of CRT, several large landmark randomised controlled trials have shown incontrovertibly that CRT leads to significant symptom improvement, reduces hospitalisations, improves morbidity and also significantly reduces mortality in CHF patients. This chapter traces the evolution in the evidence-base for CRT over the last two decades illustrating that whilst there were some differences in the inclusion criteria and end-points used in the various observational and randomised CRT studies, the broad consensus from several of these landmark trials has added substantial weight to the evidence base and led to the incorporation of CRT in national and international CHF treatment guidelines.

EARLY (OBSERVATIONAL STUDIES)

There were several non-randomised/observational studies albeit with relatively small numbers of patients and short duration of follow-up, that elucidated the beneficial effects of CRT [1, 2, 3, 4, 5, 6, 7, 8]. These early trials in the 1990s illustrated the beneficial effects of bi-ventricular pacing on acute LV haemodynamics [1, 2, 3], improved energy efficiency [9] and also improved glucose metabolism and perfusion [10]. One of the earliest of these studies was reported by Bakker et al, who employed biventricular pacing in 12 patients with end-stage CHF and left bundle branch block (LBBB) who had already been turned down for cardiac transplantation [11]. Biventricular pacing led to significant improvements in NYHA Class (NYHA Class improved from IV to II), functional capacity (peak VO_2 and exercise time) as well as echocardiographic parameters (less mitral regurgitation (MR), improved systolic and diastolic function). Leclercq et al assessed the acute haemodynamic effects due to biventricular pacing using a Swan-Ganz catheter and demonstrated a significant increase in cardiac index as well as decrease in pulmonary capillary wedge pressure in 18 patients with NYHA Class III or IV CHF and significant intra-ventricular conduction delay (170±37 ms), in comparison to intrinsic conduction or RV DDD pacing [1]. Both Kass et al [2] and Auricchio et al [3] showed that acute LV pacing in HF patients increased LV dP/dT and aortic pulse pressure especially by pacing at sites with maximum intra-ventricular conduction delay. Other early studies also showed improvement in echocardiographic parameters and thus reversal of LV remodelling due to CRT [5, 6]. Cazeau et al reported results from a randomised controlled, single-blinded, cross-over study of 47 patients with NYHA Class III HF and showed an improvement in 6 minute walk test (6MWT), quality of life (QoL) score, peak VO_2 uptake and HF hospitalisations [12]. Significant reduction in need for HF hospitalisations and hospital days was also shown in a small study by Braunshcweig et al [7]. The InSync study was a prospective observational multicentre study and followed up efficacy of CRT implants for 12 months in 103 HF patients with NYHA Class III or IV symptoms, LVEF<35%, QRS duration>150ms and LV end diastolic diameter (LVEDD)> 6 cm [8]. There was a significant shortening of QRS duration, improved mean NYHA class, 6 minute walk test and QoL score during follow-up. Detailed echocardiographic studies in 46 of these patients also showed that ejection fraction (EF) increased by nearly 5%, LV filling time increased (both statistically significant) and there was also a trend (statistically not significant) towards decrease in LV EDD, mitral regurgitation (MR) and inter-ventricular mechanical delay.

Due to the short duration of follow-up and small numbers of patients recruited, whilst these early studies demonstrated haemodynamic and symptomatic improvement due to CRT, they were not able to demonstrate a mortality benefit. They also suffered from other limitations such as lack of blinding and high drop out rates. In most of the early studies, the left ventricular lead was implanted epicardially requiring general anaesthesia and thoracotomy and this technique could have contributed to some of the procedure-related complications.

RANDOMISED TRIALS

The *PATH-CHF* (Pacing Therapies in Heart Failure) single-blind randomised cross-over controlled study enrolled 42 patients with NYHA Class III or IV symptoms, QRS duration≥120 msec and LVEF≤35% [13]. The results showed that CRT led to significant improvements acute haemodynamic effects (aortic pulse pressure and Dp/dT) as well as chronic end-points such as 6 minute walk test, QoL score (assessed by the Minnesota Living with Heart Failure questionnaire), NYHA Class and also reduced HF hospitalisations over a six month follow-up period .

The *MUSTIC* (Multi-site Stimulation in Cardiomyopathies) trial was a single-blind randomised, controlled crossover study which compared the effects of atrio-biventricular pacing (using a coronary sinus lead for LV pacing) for 3 months with that of inactive pacing (ventricular inhibited pacing at a basic rate of 40bpm) for a similar duration [14]. This trial included patients with NYHA Class III CHF of ischaemic or non-ischaemic aetiology, with LVEF<35%, LVEDD>6 cm, sinus rhythm and QRS duration>150 ms. 48 patients completed both phases of the study and the active pacing group showed a 23% increase in 6 minute walking distance ($p<0.001$), 32% improvement in QoL score ($p<0.001$), 66% reduction in hospitalisations due to CHF deterioration ($p<0.05$), 8% increase in peak oxygen uptake ($p<0.03$) and a significant proportion of patients preferred active pacing ($p<0.001$). It is to be noted that although CHF drug therapy included a 98% use of ACE inhibitors and diuretics, there was a far lower use of beta-blockers or aldosterone receptor blockers. The 3 month data of this trial showed no statistical difference in mortality between the two groups.

The *MIRACLE* (Multicentre InSync Randomised Clinical Evaluation) trial was the earliest of the double blinded RCTs [15, 16]. This trial included patients on optimum medical therapy (NB aldosterone receptor blockers were not part of standard treatment at this time) with NYHA Class III or IV CHF due to either ischaemic or non-ischaemic aetiologies. Other inclusion criteria were QRS duration≥130msec, LVEF≤35%, LV end-diastolic diameter≥5.5cm and a six-minute walking distance of ≤450m. 453 patients were randomised to receive CRT or no pacing and followed-up for six months. The CRT group showed significant improvements in all the primary end-points (6MWT,

NYHA class and QoL score) as early as one month after treatment. These improvements were independent of CHF aetiology, type of bundle branch block (left versus right) or base-line duration of the QRS interval. There was also an increase in EF of nearly 5%, reduction in severity of MR and reduction in LV diameter (3.5 mm decrease in LVIDD). The CRT group also had fewer hospitalisations, improved treadmill time and peak VO_2 . Mortality data was also available for another 79 randomised patients (532 patients in total) and showed a trend towards reduction in mortality (albeit statistically not significant- OR 0.74:95% CI 0.36-1.51).

The *MIRACLE ICD* trial was a double-blinded, randomised, controlled trial which analysed 369 patients who also had an indication for ICD therapy in addition to CRT (ICD and CRT on in 187 patients, ICD on but CRT off in 182 patients [17]. The other inclusion criteria were similar to that of that MIRACLE trial and the patients were followed up for a mean of 6 months. CRT treatment led to a significant improvement in two of the three primary endpoints such as quality of life and NYHA Class but there was no significant difference in 6 minute walk time. Whilst there were also significant increases due to CRT therapy on peak VO_2 and treadmill exercise duration, there were no significant differences in LV size, function, mortality or hospitalisations for CHF. The lack of improvement in 6 minute walking time due to CRT therapy differs from that seen in other CRT trials [15, 18] and also contrasts with the improvement seen in peak VO_2 and treadmill time. This discrepancy in addition to the lack of significant improvement in LV size or function could be explained by the fact that the patients in this trial were sicker than the MIRACLE cohort of patients.

The *CONTAK CD* Trial (N=490) was another double-blind, randomised, controlled trial that analysed the effects of CRT on patients eligible for ICD therapy for a follow-up duration of 6 months [18]. This trial was also one of the first trials in the US that used the "over the guidewire technique of lead implantation"[19]. Eligibility criteria other than that for ICD implant included NYHA class II to IV, left ventricular ejection fraction (LVEF) ≤35%, QRS interval ≥120 ms. Post-CRT implant, the trial design allowed optimisation of medical therapy prior to randomisation and this led to improvement in NYHA class to I/II in 263 patients. Whilst this diluted the numbers of patients in severe CHF, in contrast to the MIRACLE trials however this also offered an opportunity to study the effects of CRT in mild heart failure. The primary end-point in this trial was CHF progression (comprising a combination of factors such as hospitalisation for CHF, appropriate ICD therapy and all-cause mortality) and whilst there was a 15% reduction in CHF progression, this did not reach statistical significance even when analysed according to NYHA sub-groups. This was explained by the low event rate in the trial leading to the trial being under-powered. There was a significant improvement due to CRT in the secondary end-points studied (peak VO_2, 6 minute walk distance, quality of life and echocardiographic parameters such as LV dimensions, EF). Whilst patients with NYHA I/II did not show a significant improvement in functional capacity, interestingly there were significant reductions in LV dimensions in this sub-group suggesting that CRT could reverse CHF-induced remodelling in mild CHF as well. In contrast to the MIRACLE trials, the CONTAK CD trial employed "harder" primary end-points such as mortality, CHF hospitalisations and ventricular arrhythmias. However in common to the other 2 trials, whilst there was a trend towards mortality benefit due to CRT, this did not reach statistical significance - MIRACLE (OR,0.74 : 95% CI 0.36-1.51), MIRACLE ICD (OR, 0.85:95% CI 0.41-1.75) and CONTAK CD (OR, 0.67: 95% CI 0.31-1.48) [20]. This was likely to have been due to the relatively short duration of follow-up and was addressed by later landmark studies such as COMPANION and CARE-HF. A meta-analysis published shortly after the publication of these early randomised trials including MUSTIC, MIRACLE and CONTAK CD including 1634 patients, demonstrated that CRT reduced CHF hospitalisations by 29% (OR 0.71:95% CI, 0.53-0.96) and reduced HF mortality by 51% (OR, 0.49: 95% CI, 0.25-0.93). Whilst there was a trend towards reduction in all-cause mortality (OR, 0.77; 95% CI, 0.51-1.18), there was no significant reduction in either non-cardiac mortality or VT/VF in ICD patients [21].

These trials were followed by 2 large scale landmark trials (COMPANION and CARE-HF) that answered questions about the mortality benefit due to CRT. The *COMPANION Trial* (Comparison of Medical Therapy, Pacing and Defibrillation) was a multi-centre randomised controlled trial conducted in the United States which recruited 1520 patients with NYHA Class III or IV CHF (due to either ischaemic or non-ischaemic aetiology),LVEF≤35%, PR interval>150 msec, no clinical indication for pacing or ICD, QRS duration≥120 msec (>66% patients had LBBB) and at least one HF hospitalisation during the preceding year [22]. Participants were randomised in a 1:2:2 ratio to three treatment arms -optimal pharmacological therapy (OPT) alone (308 patients) versus that in combination with CRT (617 patients) or in combination with CRTD (595 patients). In contrast to previous CRT trials, OPT in this trial also included spironolactone (used in just over 50% of the patients), in addition to beta-blockers (used in about two-thirds of patients), ACE-inhibitors or ARB (used in about 90% of patients) and diuretics. Majority of the patients in the 3 treatment arms (>80%) were in NYHA Class III The primary end-point of this trial was a composite of death from any cause or hospitalisation due to any cause from the time of randomisation to the time of first event. Secondary end-point was death from any cause. Due to lack of blinding and commercial availability or both CRT pacemakers as well CRTD, the OPT treatment arm suffered the highest drop-out rate in favour of device therapy, with one in four patients dropping out and thus this group of patients had the least duration of follow-up (median follow-up 11.9 months for primary end-point) in comparison to other treatment arms. When compared to OPT, CRT (hazard ratio, 0.81; P=0.014) as well as CRTD individually reduced the risk of the primary endpoint by about 20% (hazard ratio, 0.80; P=0.01). When compared to OPT, cardiac-resynchronization therapy resulted in a 34% reduction in risk of death or hospitalisation for HF (hazard ratio, 0.66; 95% CI, 0.53 to 0.87; P<0.002), whereas CRTD reduced this risk by 40 % (hazard ratio, 0.60; 95 % CI, 0.49 to 0.75;P<0.001). Whilst there was a 24% reduction in the secondary end-point of death due to any cause, this result did not reach statistical significance (hazard ratio, 0.76; 95 percent confidence interval, 0.58 to 1.01; hazard ratio, 0.64; 95 percent confidence interval, 0.48 to 0.86;p=0.059). This was likely to have resulted from the fact that the COMPANION trial was not designed or powered to demonstrate all-cause mortality reduction by CRT alone. In comparison, CRTD significantly reduced the incidence of death due to any cause by 36% (p=0.003). In agreement with previous trials, CRT also demonstrated significant improvements in other outcome variables such as the NYHA class, the distance walked in six minutes, QoL (assessed by the Minnesota Living with Heart Failure questionnaire) and median changes in systolic blood pressure.

The *Cardiac Resynchronisation- Heart Failure (CARE-HF*) Trial was a randomised trial that enrolled 813 patients from 82 European centres [34]. Similar to the COMPANION trial CARE-HF was not a blinded study either. Inclusion criteria were comparable to those used in the COMPANION Trial (NYHA Class III or IV CHF symptoms despite OPT, LVEF≤35LVEDD, QRS duration>150msec) with the important exception of eligibility also if QRS duration was 120-150 msec along with demonstration of echocardiographic evidence of mechanical dyssynchrony (satisfying two of three additional criteria for dyssynchrony: an aortic pre-ejection delay of more than 140 msec, an interventricular mechanical delay of more than 40 msec, or delayed activation of the postero-lateral left ventricular wall). Patients with QRS duration of >150 msec constituted the majority (89%) of recruited patients.

409 CHF patients were randomised to the OPT only group and 404 were randomised to the OPT plus CRT group. The primary end point was a composite of death from any cause or an unplanned hospitalization for a major cardiovascular event. Secondary end-points assessed in the trial included mortality due to any cause, a composite of death from any cause and unplanned hospitalization with CHF, change in NYHA Class and quality of life (using Minnesota Living with Heart Failure questionnaire and European Quality of Life–5 Dimensions instrument. Other variables assessed included echocardiographic characteristics such as severity of dyssynchrony, left ventricular function, mitral regurgitation and bio-markers such as N-terminal pro–brain natriuretic peptide. Changes in heart rate and blood pressure from base-line were also recorded at follow-up. The duration of follow-up was more than double that achieved by the COMPANION trial (mean of 29.4 months). Use of beta-blockers was marginally higher (72%) than that in the COMPANION Trial (about 66%), ACE-inhibitors or ARBs 95% in CARE-HF versus about 90% in COMPANION, spironolactone use was similar (about 50-55%).

The CRT plus OPT group demonstrated a significant (37%) reduction in the primary end-point in comparison to OPT alone (55% vs 39% hazard ratio, 0.63; 95 percent confidence interval, 0.51 to 0.77; P<0.001) and 36% reduction in deaths from any cause (20% vs. 30%; hazard ratio, 0.64; 95 percent confidence interval, 0.48 to 0.85; P<0.002). CRT also demonstrated a significant reduction in the secondary end-point of risk of the composite end point of death from any cause or hospitalization for worsening heart failure (hazard ratio, 0.54; 95 percent confidence interval, 0.43 to 0.68; P<0.001). In addition there were sustained and statistically significant improvements in symptoms, quality of life, LVEF and systolic bloods pressure, echocardiographic parameters of mechanical dyssynchrony, lesser MR, left ventricular end-systolic volume index and plasma levels of NT-pro BNP. The CARE-HF trial was a landmark trial in many respects as it was the first trial to demonstrate a significant reduction in all-cause mortality due to CRT alone and also showed that the benefits of CRT extend well beyond 1 year (to 18 months). However, whilst CRT alone showed a significant improvement in all-cause mortality, a significant cause of mortality in the CRT-subgroup was due to sudden death in both trials (in about a third of patients). It can be argued that ICD therapy could have prevented most of these deaths. In addition, there is a significant overlap between the criteria used for CRT or ICD implant and CRT alone has not been shown to reduce the incidence of serious ventricular arrhythmias [17, 18, 22]. In view of all these, ICD implant adds an incremental survival advantage over and above CRT alone. CARE-HF also showed improvement in serum neuro-hormonal markers which can thus be used as another objective measure of the effectiveness of CRT. In addition, by employing the use of echocardiographic measures of mechanical dyssynchrony in the inclusion criteria, this study extended the use of CRT to patients with borderline prolonged QRS duration. It is important to note that some of the differing results between these two trials can be explained by the differences in the study populations. For instance the higher 1 year mortality in the COMPANION trial (19% versus about 13% in CARE-HF) could be explained by the fact that the COMPANION population was sicker (with a lower mean LVEF, more patients with NYHA Class IV symptomatic status and a greater proportion of patients with coronary artery disease).

In the last 5 years, 3 trials (REVERSE, RAFT and MADIT-CRT) have reported on the issue of use of CRT in patients with mild heart failure to prevent deterioration into moderate to severe heart failure. Prior to these, two other trials provided information on the effect of CRT on patients with NYHA Class 2 HF. The MIRACLE-ICD trial included 186 patients with NYHA Class 2 symptoms and during a 6 month follow-up did not show significant improvements in the primary end-point peak VO2 or in other parameters such as NYHA Class and quality of life but showed improvements in LVEF and decreased LV volumes.

CRT in Patients with Mild to Moderate Symptoms

In the last 5 years, 3 trials (REVERSE, RAFT and MADIT-CRT) have reported on the issue of use of CRT in patients with mild heart failure to prevent deterioration into moderate to severe heart failure. Prior to these, two other trials provided information on the effect of CRT on patients with NYHA Class 2 HF. The *MIRACLE-ICD* trial included 186 patients with NYHA Class 2 symptoms and during a 6 month follow-up did not show significant improvements in the primary end-point peak VO2 or in other parameters such as NYHA Class and quality of life but showed improvements in LVEF and decreased LV volumes [23].

REVERSE (Resynchronisation reverses Remodelling in Systolic left vEntricular dysfunction) Trial was a randomised double-blind trial of heart failure patients from North America and Europe with NYHA Class 1 (18%) or Class 2 (18%) including 419 patients with CRT turned on (82% of these also had an ICD) and 191 patients with CRT turned off [24]. Other inclusion criteria were LVEF≤40%, LVEDD≥55mm and QRS duration≥120ms. During the follow-up of 1 (North American centres) to 2 years (European centres), whilst CRT did not significantly reduce the primary end-point (composite of death, hospitalisation or worsening NYHA class), it led to significant reductions in CHF hospitalisations as well as time to first heart failure hospitalisation (53% relative risk reduction). CRT also led to significant reverse remodelling in the form of reduced LV volume indices and increased LVEF. These improvements were mainly driven by the sub-set of patients with QRS duration>152 msec. Importantly, approximately 95% of the patients in this trial were on both beta-blockers and ACE-inhibitors or ARBs and thus the improvements in reverse remodelling and morbidity seen in this trial were in addition to that produced by OPT. Improvements in reverse remodelling were also demonstrated in a similar cohort of patients with NYHA Class 2 symptoms even with a short duration of follow-up [18, 23]. Increased reverse remodelling also correlated with significantly lower incidence of ventricular arrhythmias. However, there were no significant improvements in either 6MWT or QoL and this could be explained by the fact that these were patients who were asymptomatic or with mild symptoms to prior to CRT. Interestingly the European cohort of patients who had a longer duration of follow-up of 2 years showed a significant improvement in the primary end-point with CRT though mortality reduction did not reach statistical significance.

The *MADIT-CRT* trial was a larger trial compared to REVERSE, enrolling 1820 patients (North America and Europe -110 centres) in a 3:2 ratio comparing effects of CRTD (1089 patients) with those of ICD only (731 patients) followed up for 2.4 years [25]. This trial also enrolled patients with NYHA Class 1 (15% of patients) or 2 but with lower LVEF (≤30%) compared to REVERSE. QRS width had to be≥130 ms and the patients were also required to have a primary prevention indication for ICD. Majority of patients were in NYHA Class 2 status (>80%), average EF was 24±5% QRS duration was significantly prolonged (>150ms in about two-thirds of patients. There was a significant reduction (34%, HR 0.66) in the primary end-point of death or heart failure in the CRTD group. This was driven mainly by the 41% decrease in heart failure events as mortality reduction was not statistically significant. The beneficial effects of CRTD were more marked amongst women, patients with LBBB or QRS duration≥150 msec although the study was not statistically powered to evaluate sub-groups. However these effects were similar irrespective of whether the HF aetiology was ischaemic or non-ischaemic. Similar to REVERSE results, MADIT-CRT also showed significantly higher reverse remodelling due to CRT as well as reduced BNP but no changes in quality of life or 6 minute walk test. The incidence of VT/VF was also similar in the two groups. A recently published cost-effectiveness study of this trial showed that CRTD was cost-effective in patients with LBBB with $58330/quality-adjusted life years CRTD vs.ICD over a 4 year period [26]. A retrospective analysis of QoL measures showed that the CRTD group of patients experienced a significant improvement vs. ICD group in patients with LBBB [27].

The *RAFT* trial [28] was another large trial which recruited 1800 patients (nearly 80% NYHA Class 2, 20% Class 3) and showed that CRTD in comparison with ICD led to a significant reduction (25%) in the primary outcome (death or hart failure). This effect was again mainly due to significant reduction in HF events as mortality reduction was not statistically significant. Indices of reverse remodelling were also significantly affected by CRT. Whilst the benefits of CRT were comparable between patients in Class 2 and Class 3, benefits were not seen in patients with RBBB or if QRS duration was ≤150 ms.

CRT in Patients with AF and Heart Failure

Atrial fibrillation can occur in one in four patients with chronic heart failure and has been shown to worsen prognosis irrespective of LV systolic function [29, 30]. The PAVE (Post-AV node ablation evaluation study compared a RV pacing strategy versus CRT in patients undergoing AV node ablation for the management of AF compared RV pacing (n=81) only versus CRT (n=103), found that 6 months post-ablation the CRT group had a significant improvement in 6 minute walk distance as well as ejection fraction especially in patients with baseline NYHA Class 2/3 status or LVEF<45% [31]. A prospective multi-centre study by Brignole et al evaluated a similar strategy did not show a mortality benefit from CRT,but the CRT group had significantly lower HF hospitalisations and worsening of HF irrespective of baseline QRS duration (≥120 ms or not) and LEVF (≤35% or not) [32]. A meta-analysis of twenty three observational studies that included nearly 1900 patients with AF who underwent CRT showed that AF increased the relative risk of all-cause mortality by 50% and the relative risk of CRT non-response by 32% [33]. AF also led to poorer functional capacity, QoL scores and LV volume. This meta-analysis suggested that AV node ablation can improve both HF outcomes as well as mortality in these patients.

CONCLUSION

CRT has been demonstrated to significantly reduce all-cause mortality, morbidity due to HF as well as echocardiographic parameters in patients with NYHA Class 3 or 4 in the landmark CARE-HF and COMPANION trials. More recent trials such as REVERSE, MADIT-CRT and RAFT have also shown that CRT could play an important role even in patients with mild HF (NYHA Class 1 or 2) by significantly reducing HF events as well as improving reverse remodelling. These effects can have an important role in preventing or delaying progression of HF. Since there is a significant overlap in the eligibility criteria for CRT or ICD, and patients with CRT only are still at significant risk of sudden arrhythmic death, combining ICD implant along with CRT is considered prudent even in patients with mild symptoms.

REFERENCES

[1] Leclercq C, Cazeau S, Le BH, et al. Acute hemodynamic effects of biventricular DDD pacing in patients with end-stage heart failure. *J. Am. Coll Cardiol.* 1998 Dec;32(7):1825-31.

[2] Kass DA, Chen CH, Curry C, et al. Improved left ventricular mechanics from acute VDD pacing in patients with dilated cardiomyopathy and ventricular conduction delay. *Circulation* 1999 Mar 30;99(12):1567-73.

[3] Auricchio A, Stellbrink C, Block M, et al. Effect of pacing chamber and atrioventricular delay on acute systolic function of paced patients with congestive heart failure. The Pacing Therapies for Congestive Heart Failure Study Group. The Guidant Congestive Heart Failure Research Group. *Circulation* 1999 Jun 15;99(23):2993-3001.

[4] Leclercq C, Cazeau S, Ritter P, et al. A pilot experience with permanent biventricular pacing to treat advanced heart failure. *Am. Heart J.* 2000 Dec;140(6):862-70.

[5] Etienne Y, Mansourati J, Touiza A, et al. Evaluation of left ventricular function and mitral regurgitation during left ventricular-based pacing in patients with heart failure. *Eur. J. Heart Fail* 2001 Aug;3(4):441-7.

[6] Lau CP, Yu CM, Chau E, et al. Reversal of left ventricular remodeling by synchronous biventricular pacing in heart failure. *Pacing Clin. Electrophysiol.* 2000 Nov;23(11 Pt 2):1722-5.

[7] Braunschweig F, Linde C, Gadler F, et al. Reduction of hospital days by biventricular pacing. *Eur. J. Heart Fail* 2000 Dec;2(4):399-406.
[8] Gras D, Leclercq C, Tang AS, et al. Cardiac resynchronization therapy in advanced heart failure the multicenter InSync clinical study. *Eur. J. Heart Fail* 2002 Jun;4(3):311-20.
[9] Nelson GS, Berger RD, Fetics BJ, et al. Left ventricular or biventricular pacing improves cardiac function at diminished energy cost in patients with dilated cardiomyopathy and left bundle-branch block. *Circulation* 2000 Dec 19;102(25):3053-9.
[10] Nowak B, Sinha AM, Schaefer WM, et al. Cardiac resynchronization therapy homogenizes myocardial glucose metabolism and perfusion in dilated cardiomyopathy and left bundle branch block. *J. Am. Coll Cardiol.* 2003 May 7;41(9):1523-8.
[11] Bakker PF, Meijburg HW, de Vries JW, et al. Biventricular pacing in end-stage heart failure improves functional capacity and left ventricular function. *J. Interv. Card Electrophysiol.* 2000 Jun;4(2):395-404.
[12] Cazeau S, Leclercq C, Lavergne T, et al. Effects of multisite biventricular pacing in patients with heart failure and intraventricular conduction delay. *N. Engl. J. Med.* 2001 Mar 22;344(12):873-80.
[13] Auricchio A, Stellbrink C, Sack S, et al. Long-term clinical effect of hemodynamically optimized cardiac resynchronization therapy in patients with heart failure and ventricular conduction delay. *J. Am. Coll. Cardiol.* 2002 Jun 19;39(12):2026-33.
[14] Linde C, Leclercq C, Rex S, et al. Long-term benefits of biventricular pacing in congestive heart failure: results from the MUltisite STimulation in cardiomyopathy (MUSTIC) study. *J. Am. Coll. Cardiol.* 2002 Jul 3;40(1):111-8.
[15] Abraham WT. Rationale and design of a randomized clinical trial to assess the safety and efficacy of cardiac resynchronization therapy in patients with advanced heart failure: the Multicenter InSync Randomized Clinical Evaluation (MIRACLE). *J. Card Fail* 2000 Dec;6(4):369-80.
[16] Abraham WT, Fisher WG, Smith AL, et al. Cardiac resynchronization in chronic heart failure. *N. Engl. J. Med.* 2002 Jun 13;346(24):1845-53.
[17] Young JB, Abraham WT, Smith AL, et al. Combined cardiac resynchronization and implantable cardioversion defibrillation in advanced chronic heart failure: the MIRACLE ICD Trial. *JAMA* 2003 May 28;289(20):2685-94.

[18] Higgins SL, Hummel JD, Niazi IK, et al. Cardiac resynchronization therapy for the treatment of heart failure in patients with intraventricular conduction delay and malignant ventricular tachyarrhythmias. *J. Am. Coll. Cardiol.* 2003 Oct 15;42(8):1454-9.

[19] Tan TC, Sindone AP, Denniss AR. Cardiac electronic implantable devices in the treatment of heart failure. *Heart Lung Circ.* 2012 Jun;21(6-7):338-51.

[20] Salukhe TV, Dimopoulos K, Francis D. Cardiac resynchronisation may reduce all-cause mortality: meta-analysis of preliminary COMPANION data with CONTAK-CD, InSync ICD, MIRACLE and MUSTIC. *Int. J. Cardiol.* 2004 Feb;93(2-3):101-3.

[21] Bradley DJ, Bradley EA, Baughman KL, et al. Cardiac resynchronization and death from progressive heart failure: a meta-analysis of randomized controlled trials. *JAMA* 2003 Feb 12;289(6):730-40.

[22] Bristow MR, Saxon LA, Boehmer J, et al. Cardiac-resynchronization therapy with or without an implantable defibrillator in advanced chronic heart failure. *N. Engl. J. Med.* 2004 May 20;350(21):2140-50.

[23] Abraham WT, Young JB, Leon AR, et al. Effects of cardiac resynchronization on disease progression in patients with left ventricular systolic dysfunction, an indication for an implantable cardioverter-defibrillator, and mildly symptomatic chronic heart failure. *Circulation* 2004 Nov 2;110(18):2864-8.

[24] Linde C, Abraham WT, Gold MR, et al. Randomized trial of cardiac resynchronization in mildly symptomatic heart failure patients and in asymptomatic patients with left ventricular dysfunction and previous heart failure symptoms. *J. Am. Coll Cardiol.* 2008 Dec 2;52(23):1834-43.

[25] Moss AJ, Hall WJ, Cannom DS, et al. Cardiac-resynchronization therapy for the prevention of heart-failure events. *N. Engl. J. Med.* 2009 Oct 1;361(14):1329-38.

[26] Noyes K, Veazie P, Hall WJ, et al. Cost-Effectiveness of Cardiac Resynchronization Therapy in the MADIT-CRT Trial. *J. Cardiovasc. Electrophysiol* 2012 Aug 22.

[27] Veazie PJ, Noyes K, Li Q, et al. Cardiac Resynchronization and Quality of Life in Patients With Minimally Symptomatic Heart Failure. *J. Am. Coll. Cardiol.* 2012 Sep 28.

[28] Tang AS, Wells GA, Talajic M, et al. Cardiac-resynchronization therapy for mild-to-moderate heart failure. *N. Engl. J. Med.* 2010 Dec 16;363(25):2385-95.

[29] Caldwell JC, Contractor H, Petkar S, et al. Atrial fibrillation is under-recognized in chronic heart failure: insights from a heart failure cohort treated with cardiac resynchronization therapy. *Europace* 2009 Oct;11(10):1295-300.

[30] Mamas MA, Caldwell JC, Chacko S, et al. A meta-analysis of the prognostic significance of atrial fibrillation in chronic heart failure. *Eur. J. Heart Fail* 2009 Jul;11(7):676-83.

[31] Doshi RN, Daoud EG, Fellows C, et al. Left ventricular-based cardiac stimulation post AV nodal ablation evaluation (the PAVE study). *J Cardiovasc Electrophysiol* 2005 Nov;16(11):1160-5.

[32] Brignole M, Botto G, Mont L, et al. Cardiac resynchronization therapy in patients undergoing atrioventricular junction ablation for permanent atrial fibrillation: a randomized trial. *Eur. Heart J.* 2011 Oct;32(19):2420-9.

[33] Wilton SB, Leung AA, Ghali WA, et al. Outcomes of cardiac resynchronization therapy in patients with versus those without atrial fibrillation: a systematic review and meta-analysis. *Heart Rhythm* 2011 Jul;8(7):1088-94.

[34] J.G.F. Cleland, J. Daubert, E. Erdmann, CARE-HF Study Investigators *et al.* The effect of cardiac resynchronization on morbidity and mortality in heart failure *N Engl J Med*, 352 (2005), pp. 1a11

Chapter 3

IDENTIFICATION OF SUITABLE CANDIDATES-GUIDELINES FOR CRT IMPLANTATION

INTRODUCTION

As discussed in the previous chapter, substantial evidence has accumulated from clinical trials and meta-analyses that support the use of cardiac resynchronisation therapy in selected individuals with heart failure (HF). Nevertheless, it remains an invasive therapy with associated risk of complications. Moreover, even when implant is successful, approximately 30% will not respond to therapy [1, 2, 3]. It is therefore important to consider carefully which patients are likely to benefit from CRT.

Guidelines regarding suitability for CRT vary between countries [4, 5, 6, 7]. This can be explained at least partly by the fact that, whilst early clinical studies identified clear categories of patients in whom benefit might be expected, subsequent examination of subgroups, and meta-analyses, have allowed extrapolation of primary outcome results into other categories. Due to various factors, including different ECG and symptomatic criteria between study participants, and the presence or absence of other cardiac conditions such as atrial fibrillation, this has resulted in several 'grey areas' of discrepancy between guidelines.

Summaries of current guidelines published by the American College of Cardiology/American Heart Association/ Heart Rhythm Society (ACC/AHA/HRS) [7] , the European Society of Cardiology [4] and a joint consensus statement by the European Heart Rhythm Association [8] (a branch of the ESC)/ HRSare shown in tables 1 and 2. In general terms, our practice is that where CRT is 'recommended' it should be offered unless there is a strongly compelling case not to proceed, while categories where CRT should be 'considered' will be influenced by multiple factors including general health and co-morbidities, patient activity levels and symptom expectations. For example, in the presence of obesity and/ or significant airways disease, improvement of dyspnoea following resynchronisation may be limited and may not justify intervention on a symptomatic basis.

For all categories of patients, it is important to emphasise that optimal medical therapy remains vital to HF management; unless there are clear contraindications, patients should have either adequate beta-blockade and angiotensin/ aldosterone blockade as pre-requisite to consideration for CRT. In addition, HF should be persistent; where functional or symptomatic recovery is expected (e.g. acute viral cardiomyopathy or following revascularisation), CRT may still be appropriate to improve symptoms and speed recovery but a decision may best be deferred until out with the acute phase.

Translating the Guidelines to Real-Life Practice

'Barn-door' Candidates (Poor LV Systolic Function, with Moderate- Severe Symptoms but Ambulant, Broad QRS Complex with LBBB Morphology)

Multiple studies and meta-analyses have demonstrated benefit in improving mortality, symptom scores and hospitalisation rates in this group [9, 10, 11]. Both American and European guidelines agree that CRT should be recommended (Class of Recommendation I) where there is poor LV function, at least moderate but not end-stage symptoms, and electrical dyssynchrony. However there are some important differences as illustrated below.

120ms or 150ms?

Dependent on the entrance criteria, clinical studies of CRT have defined 'electrical dyssynchrony' as QRS complex of either >120ms or >150ms. However, a meta-analysis combining 5 studies of CRT with around 6500 patients of all NYHA classes, suggests that clinical benefit from CRT may be limited to patients with QRS duration $\geq$ 150 msec [12].

There was a significant reduction in composite clinical end-points such as deaths and hospitalisations only amongst patients with QRS duration>150 msec (RR 0.60; 95% CI 0.53-0.67, P<0.001) in contrast to the lack of benefit amongst patients with QRS dutation 120-149 msec (RR 0.95; 95% CI 0.92-1.10, P=0.49).

Current ACC/AHA guidelines therefore restrict the strongest 'recommended' category (Class 1) for cases in which the QRS≥150ms although therapy can be considered in other cases where appropriate. The European guidelines however use a cut-off QRS duration of ≥120ms in patients with NYHA Class NYHA III, ambulatory IV symptoms and ≥130ms in patients with NYHA Class II symptoms for Class 1 recommendation of CRT implant.

Mechanical dyssynchrony on its own (i.e, in the absence of QRS prolongation) has not shown that CRT leads to clinical benefit [13] and hence CRT is not recommended for these patients in both sets of guidelines.

Type of Dyssynchrony

The MADIT-CRT, CARE-HF and RAFT studies demonstrated that the highest response rate is amongst patients with LV dyssynchrony due to LBBB [11, 14, 15], and suggest that patients with RBBB respond poorly to CRT. Other analyses have also shown a lack of evidence for benefit from CRT in patients with non-LBBB QRS morphologies [16, 17, 18]. A meta-analysis of over 5300 patients from four randomised controlled trials showed that there was a significant reduction in clinical events such as all-cause mortality and heart failure hospitalisations only amongst patients with LBBB QRS morphology (RR 0.64; 95% CI 0.52-0.77, p<0.001) in comparison to the lack of significant benefit in patients with non-LBBB QRS morphologies (RR 0.97 ;95% CI 0.82-1.15, p=0.75) [19]. This was particularly so amongst patients with RBBB (RR 0.91; 95% CI 0.69-1.2, P=0.49) or non-specific intra-ventricular conduction delay (RR1.19; 95% CI 0.87-1.63, P=0.28). However there is evidence from other studies showing benefit in patients with advanced heart failure and non-LBBB QRS morphologies only if associated with severe QRS prolongation (i.e, >150 ms) [15, 20]. There is thus consensus between both American as well as European guidelines which strongly recommend (Class 1 indication) CRT only where the widened QRS is of a LBBB morphology and non-LBBB morphologies have received weaker recommendations.

Severe (NYHA IV) Symptoms or Significant Co-Morbidities

Majority of the early CRT trials had NYHA Class 3 status and relatively few patients (approximately 10%) with NYHA Class 4 symptoms were enrolled [7]. The COMPANION study included around 200 patients with stable class IV symptoms [21].

It should be noted that these patients were stable without unscheduled hospital admissions in the month prior to study entry, and with an expected survival of at least 6 months. CRT was associated with an improved functional performance and symptom score; however, although mortality was modestly reduced it remained very high even with therapy (2 year mortality 45% vs 62% in controls). At present, guidelines do not support the use of CRT in end-stage or non-ambulatory patients with Stage D NYHA 4 HF requiring inotropes or recently-decompensated HF patients.

Poor LV, Broad QRS, Mild Symptoms

Recently, it has been proposed that early, even pre-symptomatic therapy may reverse dyssynchrony-induced ventricular remodelling and either slow or prevent heart failure progression. With this rationale, the MADIT-CRT [14], REVERSE [22], MIRACLE-ICD [23] and RAFT [15] studies have investigated whether the role of CRT should be extended to patients with mild-moderate or no symptoms (NYHA class 1 – II). Within these trials, there are echocardiographic changes suggesting left ventricular improvement, and possible benefits of slowing symptomatic progression particularly in those with widest QRS duration. CRT has shown mortality benefit amongst patients with NYHA Class II symptoms and LVEF ≤30%, but not in patients with NYHA Class 1 [15].

Based on the above results, the most significant change in the American and European guidelines has been the extension of Class 1 recommendation to include patients with NYHA Class II symptoms (NB –the 2 guidelines differ on the cut-off QRS duration and LVEF as illustrated in Tables 1and 2) [4, 7]. Patients with NYHA Class I symptoms have been given a Class IIb recommendation in the latest ACC/AHA guidelines (if LVEF≤30%, ischaemic aetiology of HF, sinus rhythm, QRS duration≥ 150 ms) whereas the European guidelines do not make similar recommendations for these patients.

Patients in Whom Conventional Pacemaker Is Indicated

There has been increasing evidence that cardiac dyssynchrony, due to pacing from the right ventricular apex, has an adverse effect on left ventricular dysfunction. The DAVID trial provided the most convincing evidence that exclusive chronic RV pacing can be detrimental especially if the total duration of pacing is ≥40% [24]. Similar results were demonstrated from the MADIT-II trial in which the cut-off for total pacing duration was >50% [25]. In light of these, where there is a conventional indication for pacemaker implantation with likelihood of significant RV pacing dependence, the new American guidelines have upgraded the class of recommendation for CRT in these patients from IIb to IIa in patients with LVEF≤35% irrespective of NYHA symptom class [7]. The European guidelines are similar in terms of the strength of recommendation except for the exclusion of patients with mild symptoms [4].

It is not uncommon for patients with advanced heart failure to develop bradycardia following initiation of beta blocker therapy. Whilst sinus bradycardia may be alleviated by a dose reduction, atrioventricular block typically heralds the presence of significant conduction system disease which is likely to worsen with heart failure progression. Given the clear symptomatic and prognostic benefit of beta blocker in all classes of heart failure, it may therefore be appropriate to consider early initiation of CRT rather than cessation of treatment.

Atrial Fibrillation

Although 25 –30 % of patients with heart failure also have AF [26] , these individuals have been under-represented in clinical studies. AF in heart failure is associated with worse symptoms, poor rate control and a poor prognosis [27]. AF in patients with CRT has also been shown to worsen outcomes [28]. Increasingly, patients with symptomatic heart failure due to impaired ejection fraction and permanent AF, have shown benefit from CRT if QRS duration is >120 ms particularly if rendered pacing dependant through AV node ablation [29, 30]. These results seem to have influenced an upgraded level of evidence (B) in the American guidelines where there class of recommendation for CRT is also stronger (IIa) than in the latest ESC guidelines (Class of recommendation IIb, Level of evidence C) [4, 7].

Table 1. 2012 ACCF/AHA/HRS/HFSA guidelines for CRT implant[7] *

Patient characteristics	Class of Recommendation*	Level of Evidence*
LVEF≤35%, sinus rhythm, LBBB with QRS duration≥150ms and NYHA III, ambulatory IV on OPT	I	A
LVEF≤35%, sinus rhythm, LBBB with QRS duration≥150ms and NYHA II	I	B
LVEF≤35%, sinus rhythm, LBBB with QRS duration=120-149ms and NYHA II, III and ambulatory IV on OPT	IIa	B
LVEF≤35%, sinus rhythm, non-LBBB pattern with QRS duration≥150ms and NYHA III/ ambulatory IV on OPT	IIa	A
LVEF≤35%, AF, on OPT and meets both following criteria 1.requirement for ventricular pacing or meets CRT criteria otherwise 2. ≈100% ventricular pacing with CRT using either rate control drugs or AV node ablation	IIa	B
Patients undergoing new or replacement pacemaker (with need for >40% ventricular pacing) with LVEF≤35% on OPT	IIa	C
LVEF≤30%, ischaemic cardiomyopathy, sinus rhythm, LBBB with QRS≥150ms, NYHA Class I on OPT	IIb	C
LVEF≤35%, sinus rhythm, non-LBBB morphology with QRS 120-149 ms, NYHA III/ ambulatory IV on OPT	IIb	B
LVEF≤35%, sinus rhythm, non-LBBB morphology with QRS ≥150ms , NYHA II on OPT	IIb	B
NYHA Class I/ II and non-LBBB morphology with QRS<150ms	III	B
Any of above if co-morbidities or frailty reduce survival to<1year	III	C

Table 2. Summary of ESC Guidelines[4] and HRA/HRS Expert Consensus Statement [8]* - 2012

Patients are considered for CRT implant if they are expected to survive for >1 year with good functional status

CLASS 1

- CRTP/CRTD in patients with LVEF≤35%, NYHA III/ ambulatory IV on OPT, sinus rhythm, LBBB QRS morphology and duration≥120ms (Level of Evidence A)
- CRT(preferably CRTD), in LVEF<30%, NYHA II despite OPT, sinus rhythm, LBBB QRS morphology and duration≥130ms (Level of Evidence A)

CLASS IIa

- CRTP/CRTD in patients with LVEF≤35%, NYHA III/ ambulatory IV on OPT, sinus rhythm, with non-LBBB QRS morphology, with QRS duration≥150ms (Level of Evidence A)
- CRT(preferably CRTD), in LVEF<30%, NYHA II despite OPT, sinus rhythm, irrespective of QRS morphology, with QRS duration≥≥150ms (Level of Evidence A)

Patients with permanent AF and LVEF≤35%, NYHA III/ ambulatory IV on OPT, sinus rhythm, LBBB QRS morphology and duration≥120ms- CRTP/CRTD may be considered (CLASS IIb, Level of evidence C)
if

1. Patient requires pacing due to intrinsically slow ventricular rate
2. Patient's ventricular rate is ≤60bpm at rest and ≤90 bpm on exercise
3. Pacemaker dependence due to AV node ablation

Patients who require conventional pacing but who otherwise would not need CRT

- CRT should be considered if NYHA III/ IV with LVEF≤35% irrespective of QRS duration to reduce risk of worsening HF (Class IIa, Level of Evidence C)
- CRT may be considered if NYHA II with LVEF≤35% irrespective of QRS duration to reduce risk of worsening HF (Class IIb, Level of Evidence C)

* Interpretation of Strength of Recommendations

Class

Class I: Intervention is useful and effective

Class IIa: Weight of evidence/opinion is in favor of usefulness/efficacy

Class IIb: Usefulness/efficacy less well-established by evidence/opinion

Class III: Intervention is not useful/effective and may be harmful

Level of Evidence

A: Sufficient evidence from multiple randomized trials

B: Limited evidence from single, randomized trial or other nonrandomized studies

C: Based on expert opinion, case studies, or standard of care

REFERENCES

[1] Auricchio A, Prinzen FW. Non-responders to cardiac resynchronization therapy: the magnitude of the problem and the issues. *Circ. J.* 2011;75(3):521-7.

[2] Zaca V, Mondillo S, Gaddi R, et al. Profiling cardiac resynchronization therapy patients: responders, non-responders and those who cannot respond--the good, the bad and the ugly? *Int. J. Cardiovasc. Imaging* 2011 Jan;27(1):51-7.

[3] Fox DJ, Fitzpatrick AP, Davidson NC. Optimisation of cardiac resynchronisation therapy: addressing the problem of "non-responders". *Heart* 2005 Aug;91(8):1000-2.

[4] McMurray JJ, Adamopoulos S, Anker SD, et al. ESC Guidelines for the diagnosis and treatment of acute and chronic heart failure 2012: The Task Force for the Diagnosis and Treatment of Acute and Chronic Heart Failure 2012 of the European Society of Cardiology. Developed in collaboration with the Heart Failure Association (HFA) of the ESC. *Eur J. Heart Fail* 2012 Aug;14(8):803-69.

[5] Barnett D, Phillips S, Longson C. Cardiac resynchronisation therapy for the treatment of heart failure: NICE technology appraisal guidance. *Heart* 2007 Sep;93(9):1134-5.

[6] Daubert JC, Saxon L, Adamson PB, et al. 2012 EHRA/HRS expert consensus statement on cardiac resynchronization therapy in heart failure: implant and follow-up recommendations and management: A registered branch of the European Society of Cardiology (ESC), and the Heart Rhythm Society; and in collaboration with the Heart Failure Society of America (HFSA), the American Society of Echocardiography (ASE), the American Heart Association (AHA), the European Association of Echocardiography (EAE) of the ESC and the Heart Failure Association of the ESC (HFA). * Endorsed by the governing bodies of AHA, ASE, EAE, HFSA, HFA, EHRA, and HRS. *Europace* 2012 Sep;14(9):1236-86.

[7] Tracy CM, Epstein AE, Darbar D, et al. 2012 ACCF/AHA/HRS Focused Update of the 2008 Guidelines for Device-Based Therapy of Cardiac Rhythm Abnormalities: A Report of the American College of Cardiology Foundation/American Heart Association Task Force on Practice Guidelines. *Heart Rhythm* 2012 Oct;9(10):1737-53.

[8] Daubert JC, Saxon L, Adamson PB, et al. 2012 EHRA/HRS expert consensus statement on cardiac resynchronization therapy in heart

failure: implant and follow-up recommendations and management. *Heart Rhythm* 2012 Sep;9(9):1524-76.

[9] Bradley DJ, Bradley EA, Baughman KL, et al. Cardiac resynchronization and death from progressive heart failure: a meta-analysis of randomized controlled trials. *JAMA* 2003 Feb 12;289(6):730-40.

[10] Salukhe TV, Francis DP, Sutton R. Comparison of medical therapy, pacing and defibrillation in heart failure (COMPANION) trial terminated early; combined biventricular pacemaker-defibrillators reduce all-cause mortality and hospitalization. *Int. J. Cardiol.* 2003 Feb;87(2-3):119-20.

[11] Cleland JG, Daubert JC, Erdmann E, et al. The effect of cardiac resynchronization on morbidity and mortality in heart failure. *N. Engl. J. Med* 2005 Apr 14;352(15):1539-49.

[12] Sipahi I, Carrigan TP, Rowland DY, et al. Impact of QRS duration on clinical event reduction with cardiac resynchronization therapy: meta-analysis of randomized controlled trials. *Arch. Intern. Med.* 2011 Sep 12;171(16):1454-62.

[13] Beshai JF, Grimm RA, Nagueh SF, et al. Cardiac-resynchronization therapy in heart failure with narrow QRS complexes. *N. Engl. J. Med.* 2007 Dec 13;357(24):2461-71.

[14] Moss AJ, Hall WJ, Cannom DS, et al. Cardiac-resynchronization therapy for the prevention of heart-failure events. *N. Engl. J. Med.* 2009 Oct 1;361(14):1329-38.

[15] Tang AS, Wells GA, Talajic M, et al. Cardiac-resynchronization therapy for mild-to-moderate heart failure. *N. Engl. J. Med.* 2010 Dec 16;363(25):2385-95.

[16] Bilchick KC, Kamath S, Dimarco JP, et al. Bundle-branch block morphology and other predictors of outcome after cardiac resynchronization therapy in Medicare patients. *Circulation* 2010 Nov 16;122(20):2022-30.

[17] Adelstein EC, Saba S. Usefulness of baseline electrocardiographic QRS complex pattern to predict response to cardiac resynchronization. *Am. J. Cardiol.* 2009 Jan 15;103(2):238-42.

[18] Rickard J, Kumbhani DJ, Gorodeski EZ, et al. Cardiac resynchronization therapy in non-left bundle branch block morphologies. *Pacing Clin. Electrophysiol.* 2010 May;33(5):590-5.

[19] Sipahi I, Chou JC, Hyden M, et al. Effect of QRS morphology on clinical event reduction with cardiac resynchronization therapy: meta-

analysis of randomized controlled trials. *Am. Heart J.* 2012 Feb;163(2):260-7.

[20] Rickard J, Bassiouny M, Cronin EM, et al. Predictors of response to cardiac resynchronization therapy in patients with a non-left bundle branch block morphology. *Am. J. Cardiol.* 2011 Dec 1;108(11):1576-80.

[21] Bristow MR, Saxon LA, Boehmer J, et al. Cardiac-resynchronization therapy with or without an implantable defibrillator in advanced chronic heart failure. *N. Engl. J. Med.* 2004 May 20;350(21):2140-50.

[22] Linde C, Abraham WT, Gold MR, et al. Randomized trial of cardiac resynchronization in mildly symptomatic heart failure patients and in asymptomatic patients with left ventricular dysfunction and previous heart failure symptoms. *J. Am. Coll. Cardiol.* 2008 Dec 2;52(23):1834-43.

[23] Abraham WT, Young JB, Leon AR, et al. Effects of cardiac resynchronization on disease progression in patients with left ventricular systolic dysfunction, an indication for an implantable cardioverter-defibrillator, and mildly symptomatic chronic heart failure. *Circulation* 2004 Nov 2;110(18):2864-8.

[24] Sharma AD, Rizo-Patron C, Hallstrom AP, et al. Percent right ventricular pacing predicts outcomes in the DAVID trial. *Heart Rhythm* 2005 Aug;2(8):830-4.

[25] Steinberg JS, Fischer A, Wang P, et al. The clinical implications of cumulative right ventricular pacing in the multicenter automatic defibrillator trial II. *J. Cardiovasc. Electrophysiol.* 2005 Apr;16(4):359-65.

[26] Caldwell JC, Contractor H, Petkar S, et al. Atrial fibrillation is under-recognized in chronic heart failure: insights from a heart failure cohort treated with cardiac resynchronization therapy. *Europace* 2009 Oct;11(10):1295-300.

[27] Mamas MA, Caldwell JC, Chacko S, et al. A meta-analysis of the prognostic significance of atrial fibrillation in chronic heart failure. *Eur. J. Heart Fail* 2009 Jul;11(7):676-83.

[28] Wilton SB, Leung AA, Ghali WA, et al. Outcomes of cardiac resynchronization therapy in patients with versus those without atrial fibrillation: a systematic review and meta-analysis. *Heart Rhythm* 2011 Jul;8(7):1088-94.

[29] Brignole M, Botto G, Mont L, et al. Cardiac resynchronization therapy in patients undergoing atrioventricular junction ablation for permanent

atrial fibrillation: a randomized trial. *Eur. Heart J.* 2011 Oct; 32(19):2420-9.

[30] Wilton SB, Leung AA, Ghali WA, et al. Outcomes of cardiac resynchronization therapy in patients with versus those without atrial fibrillation: a systematic review and meta-analysis. *Heart Rhythm* 2011 Jul; 8(7):1088-94.

Chapter 4

Implant Technique

Introduction

Early studies of cardiac resynchronisation therapy (CRT) involved conventional transvenous implantation of right atrial (RA) and right ventricular (RV) leads, with an epicardial left ventricular (LV) lead being placed thorascopically or via thoracotomy [1, 2].

This technique has several disadvantages, including a requirement for general anaesthesia, prolonged hospital stay and significant morbidity and mortality.

Moreover, the long-term electrical properties of epicardial electrodes have proven to be sub-optimal, with a high incidence of late lead failure due to exit block [3].

Complete transvenous implantation of CRT systems was first reported in 1998 [4]. This technique is an extension of conventional pacing systems, with the addition of an extra lead which is placed via a catheter in the coronary sinus (CS) and positioned in a suitable epicardial vein draining the LV free wall.

Subsequently, with rapid development of the technique and equipment, this has become the preferred approach and successful implant can be achieved in >90% of patients with a low incidence of major complications [5]. With experience, most operators will develop their own techniques and tricks. The following should not be considered to be a description of 'the ideal implant technique', but rather some tips and techniques based on the authors' own experiences in addition to those suggested by international guidelines [5, 6].

KEY STEPS TO A SUCCESSFUL IMPLANT

- Prepare the patient and equipment
- Fashion the generator pocket
- Gain vascular access
- Implant RV and RA leads (RA lead can be omitted if there is permanent AF)
- Access the CS with guide catheter
- Perform contrast fluoroscopy to assess anatomy
- Position LV lead in a suitable branch
- Ensure lead parameters are satisfactory; split and remove guide catheter
- Secure leads, attach generator and close the wound

PRE-IMPLANT CONSIDERATIONS

- A detailed history should be elicited including co-morbidities and assessment of approximate life expectancy
- Physical examination is essential with particular focus on heart failure (HF) status
- Assessment of functional status using tests such as 6 minute walk test and assessment of quality of life scores have been used as tools of a multi-pronged strategy (mainly as secondary end-points) in order to evaluate success of CRT in trials (refer Chapter 2). These require a pre-implant evaluation and repeat assessments post-implant at three to six monthly intervals for a certain period of time. Whilst the applicability of these in real life practice has not been widespread, they certainly offer a valuable method of objectively quantifying change in morbidity due to therapy.
- Evaluation of HF aetiology (ischaemic vs. non-ischaemic) using coronary angiography or non-invasive tests (stress echocardiography, nuclear imaging or stress CMR) can help identify patients who require revascularisation or identify viable myocardium and thus help direct LV lead implantation strategies.
- Ensuring optimum HF drug therapy and stability for at least 3 months prior to implant [5]

- Similar to any other pre-operative work-up, baseline blood tests including complete haemogram, renal function, liver function, coagulation profile and serum glucose levels, are indicated. Chest X-Ray and pulmonary function testing are useful to assess for significant lung disease which may dilute the symptomatic benefits of CRT. CRT trials have shown that levels of natriuretic peptides such as BNP and NT-proBNP are reduced post-implant and hence assessing these pre-implant could be useful [7, 8].Up-to-date 12 lead ECG and detailed echocardiogram should be performed to assess LV ejection fraction (LVEF), cardiac dimensions and valvular function. Whilst pre-implant imaging for mechanical dyssynchrony can be useful in patients with borderline QRS duration, it should not be used on its own to exclude patients from consideration of CRT implant.
- It is especially important to plan a clear strategy regarding the pre-implant and post-implant dosing regimen for patients on anti-coagulants. In patients with low to moderate thrombo-embolic risk, the implanting physician has to balance the risk-versus benefits of stopping anti-coagulants 3-5 days prior implant or modifying dose to maintain INR 1.5-2.5 [5]. Amongst patients with a high thrombo-embolic risk, the recommendation is to continue warfarin whilst maintaining INR between 2-3 [5].

IMPLANT CONSIDERATIONS

- In the vast majority of cases, implantation can be performed safely under conscious sedation and local anaesthesia even when a combined pacemaker-defibrillator is utilised [9]. It is important to be aware however that these are patients with a fragile haemodynamic balance which can be tilted by hypotension (due to use of sedation), dehydration (due to a combination of pre-operative fasting and prolonged procedure times) and risk of respiratory depression (due to use of intravenous sedation and opiate analgesia). Careful haemodynamic monitoring and attention to volume status are thus paramount.
- Typical procedure times are under 120 minutes [10], during which time the patient will be lying supine. However, due to the unpredictable nature of coronary sinus anatomy, in complex cases the

duration may far exceed this, thus increasing the risks of dehydration or pulmonary oedema

- General anaesthesia may be appropriate for very young or restless patients, or where co-morbidities such as obesity, respiratory disease or haemodynamic instability preclude safe use of conscious sedation. Where possible, potential problems should be anticipated and anaesthesiology opinion sought early.
- Due to the prolonged procedure times, the risk of infection exceeds that of conventional pacemaker procedures. Strict sterile precautions are mandatory; where possible implants should be performed in a dedicated 'clean' operating theatre. Antibiotic prophylaxis decreases the risk of device infection and is recommended by the latest ACC/AHA/HRS as well as EHRA guidelines [5, 11].
- Adequate high quality fluoroscopic imaging is necessary, including a 'roadmap' screen to display saved images. Although not essential, a biplane system allows easier visualisation of coronary sinus anatomy.
- Previous coronary angiography images should be reviewed prior to implant as they may demonstrate late phase coronary venous drainage for localisation of the coronary sinus.
- If the patient has a previous pacing system, a peripheral venogram should be performed to ensure vessel patency. Occluded or stenosed vessels may require specialised techniques including balloon dilatation, lead extraction or contralateral lead implant, all of which greatly increase procedure complexity.
- Patients with complex congenital cardiac anatomy should not undergo implantation without a thorough understanding of the venous anatomy; 3D imaging techniques such as CT or MRI are invaluable in this setting.
- In the authors' experience, dual anti-platelet therapy is associated with more significant bleeding problems and where possible implantation should be delayed if this cannot be interrupted.

Equipment for CRT Implant

- Standard equipment for conventional pacing system implantation
    - Selection of RA and RV leads

- o Percutaneous sheaths for lead introduction
- o Appropriate surgical equipment for pocket formation, including toothed and non-toothed forceps, self-retaining retractors, large and small vessel clips

- – Contrast agent for coronary sinus venography (make sure the patient is hydrated!)
- – Coronary sinus guide catheters of assorted shapes, with appropriate haemostatic valves and introducer sheaths
- – J-tipped long guide wire, and assorted angioplasty guide wires
- – Occlusion balloon with injectable lumen for coronary sinus venogram
- – Selection of LV leads of different calibres and fixation types

General Approach to Implant Procedure

- – A left sided implant is usually easiest. As modern generators are small and unobtrusive, even left-handed patients are unlikely to experience disadvantage from a dominant-sided implant*. Where a combined resynchronisation/ defibrillator device is indicated, defibrillation thresholds are likely to be more reliable from the left side.
- – A left sided approach allows the leads to follow a gentle curve through the superior vena cava into the heart. Right sided implants are more difficult, as the leads must negotiate a secondary S-bend at the junction of the subclavian vein.
- – Nevertheless, the operator should gain experience in implanting from either side for cases when a left sided approach is not possible.
- – Sub-pectoral pockets provide a superior cosmetic appearance, particularly for defibrillation devices and in thin patients. However, subsequent generator replacement procedures are substantially quicker and easier with subcutaneous pockets. In the presence of scar tissue a 'simple' sub-pectoral generator change might take as long as the original implant and require general anaesthesia for patient comfort.
- – A modified Seldinger approach to the subclavian vein is normal practice due to the use of bulky sheaths to access the coronary sinus.

* In our experience, the one exception has been a left-handed shooting enthusiast whose rifle abutted the generator, resulting in a request for a contralateral repositioning.

Recently, cardiac synchronisation purely via the cephalic vein, has been shown to be feasible and safe [12].

- A peripheral venogram can be very helpful to identify venous anatomy, particularly for obese patients or those with unusual chest anatomy.

Special Considerations: Right Ventricular and Right Atrial Leads

- The RV lead should be implanted first. In patients with left bundle branch block, trauma to the right bundle branch during guide catheter manipulation can result in sudden and unpredictable complete heart block.
- Successful resynchronisation is highly dependent on the maintenance of atrio-ventricular (AV) synchrony; it is therefore necessary to implant the RA lead in a position that gives adequate sensing of atrial activity. Where a lead placed conventionally in the atrial appendage is inadequate due to low amplitude signal, a position on the lateral wall close to the sinus node may be appropriate although this increases the risk of lead displacement.
- The atrial lead can become dislodged during cannulation of the coronary sinus; for this reason some operators prefer to place this lead at the end of the procedure. However, manipulation of the atrial lead can occasionally dislodge the LV lead, resulting in a far more difficult repositioning.

Cannulation of the Coronary Sinus and Contrast Fluoroscopy

- The coronary sinus is behind the right AV groove and drains into the posterior base of the right atrium
- Cannulation is easiest using an LAO 30 – 40 projection; in this view the sinus runs posteriorly across the spine
- After the guide catheter is advanced towards the floor of the right atrium, removing the guidewire should cause the tip to orientate upwards. Subsequently, gently withdrawing with counterclockwise

rotation will point it towards the posterior wall and probing with the J wire should locate the ostium of the coronary sinus.

- It is important to remember that there are variations in the angulation and diameter of the ostium between patients [13] related to gender or ischaemic heart disease. In heart failure (especially with ischaemic aetiology), atrial dilatation may result in a coronary sinus that is lower and more posteriorly-directed than expected. Use of a catheter with a wider curve may be necessary. Patients with a history of lateral myocardial infarct also have a lower prevalence of lateral veins [13]. A prominent Thesbesian valve can also impede intubation of the ostium, requiring a more inferior and ventricular entry [14].
- If cannulation is difficult, a second narrow calibre catheter can be passed through the lumen of the guide catheter. This can be used as a telescopic system for greater manoeuvrability in initial identification of the sinus.
- After the coronary sinus is cannulated, contrast can be injected via the guide catheter. This may be sufficient to demonstrate the anatomy; if vigorous venous blood flow precludes complete vessel opacification then the coronary sinus should be occluded with a balloon and further contrast injected via the lumen. Two separate projections (usually LAO 30-40 and PA or RAO 30) will allow an appreciation of the distribution of left ventricular veins. Coronary sinus spasm, stenosis or valves(particularly the valve of Vieussens) may hinder easy advancement of the lead [14]. This can be overcome by balloon dilatation or use of stiffer guidewires and gradual lead advancement after inserting the guide catheter deeper into the CS using multiple fluoroscopic veiws.
- Coronary Dissection can result from vigorous insertion of the guide catheter at an inadequate angle, or by inflation of the occlusion balloon or cannulation of a side branch. This can be identified by the extravasation of contrast material around the guide catheter. Usually, blood is contained within the adipose tissue surrounding the vessel; in this case the contrast persists around the dissection site, there is usually no haemodynamic significance and the dissection can be crossed carefully with a wire in the true lumen. If the contrast immediately washes out into the pericardium or if the dissection is equal to or exceeds the luminal diameter of the dissected vessel("major dissection" [15]), haemodynamic compromise is more likely and the procedure will probably need to be abandoned with

careful patient monitoring, serial echocardiography and possible need for pericardiocentesis or surgical repair.

Selecting a Target Vein and Positioning LV Lead

- The best results for resynchronisation occur when the LV lead is positioned on the area of most delayed activation (usually posterior or lateral free wall in patients with LBBB). A variety of imaging studies have shown that this leads to improved LV synchrony and ejection fraction, however there is still controversy regarding the most optimum site [16, 17]. LV free wall stimulation has been shown to improve acute and short term haemodynamic performance and LV systolic performance following CRT implant [18]. Thus the LV lead is usually positioned into a lateral or postero-lateral branch as anatomically and electrically distant as possible from the RV lead. Conversely, positioning on the anterior wall or at the apex may worsen acute haemodynamic function as well as long term outcome [18, 19, 20]. Increased global scar burden and trans-mural postero-lateral scar have been shown to predict lack of response from CRT if the LV lead is implanted at a scarred area [21, 22]. CMR imaging prior to implant may be thus useful in assessing these and deciding the optimum implant site especially if there is a history of previous myocardial infarction [5].
- Where a suitable vein cannot be identified, withdrawing the guide catheter to the coronary sinus ostium may reveal a large low posterior vein extending around the apex. The target implant site can be accessed via downstream branches of the middle cardiac or anterior inter-ventricular veins [23].
- For large veins, a lead may be introduced directly via the guide catheter and steered into the appropriate branch. Smaller veins may be 'probed' gently with a soft angioplasty wire, allowing placement of a thin over-the-wire lead.
- Matching the lead calibre and shape to the target vessel allows for a more secure placement and reduces the chances of the lead dislodging. Active fixation LV lead or coronary stent placement beside the lead can be used to improve stability in case of repeated intra-procedural or post-procedure dislodgement [24, 25]. In case of

extreme branch tourtuosity, a double-wire or buddy-wire technique can be used to "straighten" the course [26].

- Bi-polar leads are usually preferred by most centres due to the increased availability of different pacing vector configurations to avoid phrenic nerve stimulation or increased pacing threshold [27]. Quadripolar leads which have come into use recently, offer more options in terms of pacing configurations [28]
- The lead should be tested thoroughly before its position is accepted. Biventricular pacing (with RV apical pacing) is usually characterised by frontal plane QRS axis in right superior quadrant and a dominant R wave in V1 [29].
- Whilst a low stimulation threshold is preferable, higher thresholds (up to 3 –4V) are manageable if no other potential target veins are apparent.
- Phrenic nerve stimulation is common (up to 37% at implant or during follow-up [30]) due to the close proximity of the LV free wall to the nerve and this poses a significant challenge to LV lead implant as well as post-procedural outcome [30]. The nerve courses close to the lateral or posterior coronary veins in over three quarters of cases [31, 32]. This should be assessed using high output (10V) during deep inspiration and expiration, whilst simultaneously palpating the patient's abdomen, assessing patient's symptoms and observing diaphragmatic movement using fluoroscopy. The stimulation threshold of the left ventricle relative to the phrenic nerve will rise when patients sit and stand post-procedure; for this reason the presence of any phrenic nerve stimulation should usually prompt an attempt at identifying a different lead position to avoid an almost-inevitable subsequent revision procedure. Alternative sites are therefore usually sought, however these sites could ultimately lead to inferior outcomes and lead dislodgement [30, 32]. Increasingly with availability of multi-electrode LV leads such as bi-polar or quadripolar LV leads that offer multiple programmable pacing vectors, the problem of phrenic nerve stimulation can be solved by changing the pacing vector [27]. By allowing the option of programming wither the distal or proximal electrode as cathode, the farthest electrode from the phrenic nerve can be used for pacing and several pacing configurations can be tried (such as LV ring to can, LV ring to RV coil, LV tip to RV coil and LV tip to ring in bipolar leads) [30].

Splitting and Removing the Guide Catheter

- Following satisfactory position of the LV lead, the guide catheter is carefully withdrawn into the right atrium and the lead stabilised with a stylet.
- With the lead held securely in a specialised cutting tool, the catheter is pulled with a single smooth movement to split along its length. Fluoroscopic guidance during this process enables simultaneous monitoring of the LV lead to ensure it doesn't get dislodged.
- Unfortunately, if the lead becomes dislodged at this point it is usually not possible to reposition it and the coronary sinus must be re-cannulated from the beginning.

Complications of CRT Implant

A recent systematic review of 7 non-thoracotomy CRT implant trials that included over 4500 patients, revealed a 7.5% incidence of failure to implant CS lead [33]. Inhospital mortality was 0.3% and 1 month mortality was 0.7% [33]. In comparison a study of nearly 31000 Medicare patients with CRT implants showed a higher in-hospital mortality of 1.1% [34]. The incidence of pneumothorax varied from 0.9% to 1.2% [33, 34] and the incidence of complications related to coronary veins was 2% (including dissection, perforation and cardiac tamponade) [33]. Rates of lead dislodgements varied from 2.9% to 10.6% and incidence of pocket haematomas requiring surgical intervention was 2.4% [33]. Early complications (including lead dislodgement and coronary sinus dissection or perforation) seen in 10 % within 24 hours , late complications (mainly lead dislodgements in 5.5% within a month in the CARE-HF Study [32]. Importantly, this review showed a steady decline in complications in the more recent trials, reflecting a combination of better technology and improved implanter experience.

Post-Implant Care and Follow-Up

- Patients are usually kept in hospital overnight after CRT implant and monitoring of baseline clinical parameters recorded.

- Routine post-implant investigations include chest xray (to exclude pneumothorax and confirm leads positions), 12 lead ECG(confirming biventricular capture) and echocardiography . Biventricular pacing (with RV apical pacing) is usually characterised by frontal plane QRS axis in right superior quadrant and a dominant R wave in V1 [29]. Absence of these features should prompt ruling out of LV lead displacement or lack of capture. Echocardiography pre-discharge can be considered to assess the acute effects of CRT and compare
- The device is usually programmed to VDD/DDD pacing mode. The AV delay is usually set at 100-120 ms and echo-based AV/VV optimisation has not been shown to improve response [5]. However an echo based AV optimisation is recommended if the mitral inflow pattern post-procedure shows sub-optimal filling pattern (i.e. stage 2 or 3 diastolic dysfunction) [35].
- Prior to discharge the pacemaker pocket is re-examined for haematoma.
- Post-implant clinic follow-up at 3/6 monthly intervals to conduct a detailed symptomatic response assessment (including quality of life score), physical examination, optimization of medical therapy and testing of device parameters. Functional testing such as 6 minute walk test or exercise test is also considered.
- Remote monitoring for arrhythmias and heart failure deterioration has been shown to be advantageous and predicts risk of hospitalisation [5].

REFERENCES

[1] Auricchio A, Stellbrink C, Sack S, et al. Long-term clinical effect of hemodynamically optimized cardiac resynchronization therapy in patients with heart failure and ventricular conduction delay. *J. Am. Coll. Cardiol.* 2002 Jun 19;39(12):2026-33.

[2] Saxon LA, Boehmer JP, Hummel J, et al. Biventricular pacing in patients with congestive heart failure: two prospective randomized trials. The VIGOR CHF and VENTAK CHF Investigators. *Am. J. Cardiol.* 1999 Mar 11;83(5B):120D-3D.

[3] Fortescue EB, Berul CI, Cecchin F, et al. Patient, procedural, and hardware factors associated with pacemaker lead failures in pediatrics and congenital heart disease. *Heart Rhythm* 2004 Jul;1(2):150-9.

[4] Daubert JC, Ritter P, Le BH, et al. Permanent left ventricular pacing with transvenous leads inserted into the coronary veins. *Pacing Clin. Electrophysiol.* 1998 Jan;21(1 Pt 2):239-45.

[5] Daubert JC, Saxon L, Adamson PB, et al. 2012 EHRA/HRS expert consensus statement on cardiac resynchronization therapy in heart failure: implant and follow-up recommendations and management. *Heart Rhythm* 2012 Sep;9(9):1524-76.

[6] Tracy CM, Epstein AE, Darbar D, et al. 2012 ACCF/AHA/HRS Focused Update of the 2008 Guidelines for Device-Based Therapy of Cardiac Rhythm Abnormalities: A Report of the American College of Cardiology Foundation/American Heart Association Task Force on Practice Guidelines. *Heart Rhythm* 2012 Oct;9(10):1737-53.

[7] Cleland JG, Freemantle N, Daubert JC, et al. Long-term effect of cardiac resynchronisation in patients reporting mild symptoms of heart failure: a report from the CARE-HF study. *Heart* 2008 Mar;94(3):278-83.

[8] Fruhwald FM, Fahrleitner-Pammer A, Berger R, et al. Early and sustained effects of cardiac resynchronization therapy on N-terminal pro-B-type natriuretic peptide in patients with moderate to severe heart failure and cardiac dyssynchrony. *Eur. Heart J.* 2007 Jul;28(13):1592-7.

[9] Fox DJ, Davidson NC, Royle M, et al. Safety and acceptability of implantation of internal cardioverter-defibrillators under local anesthetic and conscious sedation. *Pacing Clin. Electrophysiol.* 2007 Aug;30(8):992-7.

[10] Merkely B, Molnar L, Szilagyi S, et al. Advanced Techniques for CRT Implantation. In: Das MK, editor. *Modern Pacemakers - Present and Future*. InTech, 2011.

[11] Baddour LM, Epstein AE, Erickson CC, et al. Update on cardiovascular implantable electronic device infections and their management: a scientific statement from the American Heart Association. *Circulation* 2010 Jan 26;121(3):458-77.

[12] Ussen B, Dhillon PS, Anderson L, et al. Safety and feasibility of cephalic venous access for cardiac resynchronization device implantation. *Pacing Clin. Electrophysiol.* 2011 Mar;34(3):365-9.

[13] Blendea D, Shah RV, Auricchio A, et al. Variability of coronary venous anatomy in patients undergoing cardiac resynchronization therapy: a

high-speed rotational venography study. *Heart Rhythm* 2007 Sep;4(9):1155-62.

[14] Morgan JM, Delgado V. Lead positioning for cardiac resynchronization therapy: techniques and priorities. *Europace* 2009 Nov;11 Suppl 5:v22-v28.

[15] de Cock CC, van Campen CM, Visser CA. Major dissection of the coronary sinus and its tributaries during lead implantation for biventricular stimulation: angiographic follow-up. *Europace* 2004 Jan;6(1):43-7.

[16] Khan FZ, Virdee MS, Fynn SP, et al. Left ventricular lead placement in cardiac resynchronization therapy: where and how? *Europace* 2009 May;11(5):554-61.

[17] Singh JP, Mela T. Anatomical left ventricular lead location and clinical outcome: not a one size fit all strategy. *Europace* 2012 Aug;14(8):1076-8.

[18] Butter C, Auricchio A, Stellbrink C, et al. Effect of resynchronization therapy stimulation site on the systolic function of heart failure patients. *Circulation* 2001 Dec 18;104(25):3026-9.

[19] Singh JP, Klein HU, Huang DT, et al. Left ventricular lead position and clinical outcome in the multicenter automatic defibrillator implantation trial-cardiac resynchronization therapy (MADIT-CRT) trial. *Circulation* 2011 Mar 22;123(11):1159-66.

[20] Dong YX, Powell BD, Asirvatham SJ, et al. Left ventricular lead position for cardiac resynchronization: a comprehensive cinegraphic, echocardiographic, clinical, and survival analysis. *Europace* 2012 Aug;14(8):1139-47.

[21] Ypenburg C, Schalij MJ, Bleeker GB, et al. Impact of viability and scar tissue on response to cardiac resynchronization therapy in ischaemic heart failure patients. *Eur. Heart J.* 2007 Jan;28(1):33-41.

[22] Bleeker GB, Kaandorp TA, Lamb HJ, et al. Effect of posterolateral scar tissue on clinical and echocardiographic improvement after cardiac resynchronization therapy. *Circulation* 2006 Feb 21;113(7):969-76.

[23] Singh JP, Heist EK, Ruskin JN, et al. "Dialing-in" cardiac resynchronization therapy: overcoming constraints of the coronary venous anatomy. *J. Interv. Card Electrophysiol.* 2006 Oct;17(1):51-8.

[24] Luedorff G, Kranig W, Grove R, et al. Improved success rate of cardiac resynchronization therapy implant by employing an active fixation coronary sinus lead. *Europace* 2010 Jun;12(6):825-9.

[25] Geller L, Szilagyi S, Zima E, et al. Long-term experience with coronary sinus side branch stenting to stabilize left ventricular electrode position. *Heart Rhythm* 2011 Jun;8(6):845-50.

[26] Chierchia GB, Geelen P, Rivero-Ayerza M, et al. Double wire technique to catheterize sharply angulated coronary sinus branches in cardiac resynchronization therapy. *Pacing Clin. Electrophysiol.* 2005 Feb;28(2):168-70.

[27] Gurevitz O, Nof E, Carasso S, et al. Programmable multiple pacing configurations help to overcome high left ventricular pacing thresholds and avoid phrenic nerve stimulation. *Pacing Clin. Electrophysiol.* 2005 Dec;28(12):1255-9.

[28] Shetty AK, Duckett SG, Bostock J, et al. Use of a quadripolar left ventricular lead to achieve successful implantation in patients with previous failed attempts at cardiac resynchronization therapy. *Europace* 2011 Jul;13(7):992-6.

[29] Barold SS, Herweg B, Giudici M. Electrocardiographic follow-up of biventricular pacemakers. *Ann. Noninvasive Electrocardiol.* 2005 Apr;10(2):231-55.

[30] Biffi M, Moschini C, Bertini M, et al. Phrenic stimulation: a challenge for cardiac resynchronization therapy. *Circ. Arrhythm. Electrophysiol.* 2009 Aug;2(4):402-10.

[31] Sanchez-Quintana D, Cabrera JA, Climent V, et al. How close are the phrenic nerves to cardiac structures? Implications for cardiac interventionalists. *J. Cardiovasc. Electrophysiol.* 2005 Mar;16(3):309-13.

[32] Gras D, Bocker D, Lunati M, et al. Implantation of cardiac resynchronization therapy systems in the CARE-HF trial: procedural success rate and safety. *Europace* 2007 Jul;9(7):516-22.

[33] van Rees JB, de Bie MK, Thijssen J, et al. Implantation-related complications of implantable cardioverter-defibrillators and cardiac resynchronization therapy devices: a systematic review of randomized clinical trials. *J. Am. Coll. Cardiol.* 2011 Aug 30;58(10):995-1000.

[34] Reynolds MR, Cohen DJ, Kugelmass AD, et al. The frequency and incremental cost of major complications among medicare beneficiaries receiving implantable cardioverter-defibrillators. *J. Am. Coll. Cardiol.* 2006 Jun 20;47(12):2493-7.

[35] Gorcsan J, III, Abraham T, Agler DA, et al. Echocardiography for cardiac resynchronization therapy: recommendations for performance and reporting--a report from the American Society of Echocardiography

Dyssynchrony Writing Group endorsed by the Heart Rhythm Society. *J. Am. Soc. Echocardiogr.* 2008 Mar;21(3):191-213.

Chapter 5

Programming and Optimisation

General Programming Considerations

- Key aim is for 100% BiV pacing
- When in sinus rhythm, minimising atrial pacing may be beneficial
- LV lead output can be set relatively low to preserve battery life
- Lead position problems may manifest as changes in the paced QRS or as phrenic nerve stimulation
- Some devices allow 'electrical repositioning' of multipolar leads to obtain satisfactory LV stimulation

General Optimisation Consideration

- Assessment of patients should include clinical status (drugs, physical activity, symptoms), ECG and device interrogation (lead parameters, histograms, pace/ sense profiles). Some devices include impedance-based fluid status monitor which may be a useful guide but not the basis for therapy.
- Atrial arrhythmias should be treated aggressively; AV node ablation may be appropriate
- AV synchronisation may be optimised using echocardiography or automatic algorithms although long-term clinical benefit has not been demonstrated

– VV optimisation has not been shown to be effective but may be indicated in cases of complex scarring or suboptimal lead position

It is important to note that CRT device programming, like all aspects of heart failure management, affects patients in different ways. An individual patient-centred approach is therefore necessary to obtain optimal outcomes.

PROGRAMMING CONSIDERATIONS

Aim for 100% Biventricular Pacing

In conventional right ventricular pacing, high proportions of ventricular paced beats are associated with poor outcomes, with an increased risk of heart failure progression. Modern pacemakers therefore are equipped with sophisticated algorithms which aim to minimise RV pacing, for example with intermittent prolongation of A-V conduction times to search for intrinsic QRS complexes. Conversely, with CRT, the clinical response is dependent on high proportions of biventricular paced beats, replacing the intrinsic pathological ventricular activation.

As most CRT devices are programmed in DDD(+/-R) mode, a key programming decision is the selection of an appropriate A-V pacing interval. This should be shorter than the intrinsic conduction time to ensure biventricular pacing prior to the arrival of an intrinsic QRS complex. Many patients with heart failure have impaired AV nodal conduction; appropriate pacing may therefore be achieved with a 'physiological' A-V interval. However, in individuals with normal AV conduction, it is necessary to ensure a balance between pacing with an A-V interval that is sufficiently short to ensure appropriate ventricular activation, but not so short as to compromise ventricular diastolic filling (see below).

Appropriate Atrial Tracking

In normal sinus rhythm, ventricular pacing which is driven by sensed intrinsic atrial activity appears to be associated with improved haemodynamics and a reduced risk of AF compared to sequential atrio-ventricular pacing. CRT devices should therefore be programmed with an upper tracking rate suitable for the expected physiological range (for example at a rate≈80% of maximal age-predicted heart rate [1]), which may include episodes of rapid sinus tachycardia during exertion. There is no general consensus for the optimal minimum heart rate in patients with heart failure, particularly when drug therapy includes beta blockers. Increasing the pacemaker lower tracking rate (the rate at which atrial pacing will commence) from 40bpm to 70bpm increases cardiac output through chronotropic mechanisms but without increasing stroke volume. In asymptomatic patients, lower tracking rate may be appropriate, but where there are symptoms to suggest concurrent sinus node dysfunction, these may be alleviated by increasing the rate and enabling sensor-driven rate response algorithms.

LEFT VENTRICULAR LEAD PROGRAMMING

With conventional pacemakers for bradycardic indications, it is usual to program a pacing output of at least double the lead stimulation threshold in order to maintain a safety margin and prevent catastrophic pacing failure. The situation with biventricular pacemakers differs in two key aspects. Firstly, although failure to capture LV pacing impulses will compromise clinical benefit, it will not cause life-threatening bradycardia in the presence of a functioning RV lead. Secondly, LV leads often have higher pacing thresholds; a conventional safety margin can require substantial output currents, causing rapid battery drain and risking phrenic nerve stimulation. Consequently, the LV lead can be programmed with a stimulation output only slightly higher (1.3 – 1.5 times) than the threshold required for capture. If low stimulation outputs are used, it is essential to test device function with the patient both supine and upright to ensure no positional failure to capture. Any pacing system requires two electrodes for delivery of a pacing stimulus. Unipolar LV leads allow limited selection of pacing configuration, with either the RV lead or the generator can be used as the second electrode. Conversely, bipolar or quadripolar leads and modern generators allow for the selection of multiple different LV pacing vectors, using either or both LV lead electrodes, as well as RV lead electrodes and, where present, defibrillator coils.

RECOGNISING AND TREATING LV LEAD PROBLEMS

Problems with the LV lead typically take the form of failure to capture, or symptomatic phrenic nerve stimulation (diaphragmatic twitch). These can be considered in terms of the relative thresholds required to stimulate myocardium compared to the phrenic nerve, which passes close to the LV free wall. Unfortunately, the optimum lead positions for cardiac benefit from CRT correspond closely with the likelihood for phrenic nerve stimulation, and this remains a major limitation in delivering effective CRT. Changes in thresholds can result from lead movement, (which may or may not be visible on X-Ray), lead maturation, or the positioning of the lead over an area of scar tissue.

Failed LV capture may manifest clinically as a modest deterioration in patient symptoms, which might be missed without specific questioning but should be apparent on 12 lead ECG as a change in the QRS axis and morphology. Modern generators can be programmed to identify loss of capture by analysing the intra-cardiac electrogram, and automatically increase output to compensate; this increase in output may cause phrenic nerve stimulation as a presenting symptom. Nevertheless, where LV lead problems are suspected, a 12 lead ECG should be performed in a variety of patient positions and with deep inspiration.

In many cases, suboptimal LV function can be resolved by judicious programming of the pacing vector, output voltage and stimulation pulse width. However, whilst it is usually possible to achieve reliable LV lead capture, where this cannot be obtained below the phrenic nerve stimulation threshold then a lead revision procedure is indicated.

Optimising Response to CRT

Following commencement of CRT, the majority of patients experience clinical improvement within 3 – 6 months. Although there is undoubtedly a strong placebo effect following device implantation, clinical studies demonstrate robust improvements in object measures on echocardiography and exercise capacity testing. The post-implant follow-up should be considered to be an ideal opportunity to initiate a comprehensive assessment and optimise therapy. However, in order to maintain and enhance benefit, this process should be continued throughout the patient's ongoing therapy and particularly when there are changes in the clinical circumstances.

Whilst this will involve assessment and alterations of device function, it is important to note that CRT optimisation should involve assessment of the overall condition, including drug therapy. For example, the device may indicate the presence of paroxysmal AF which may warrant anticoagulation, or it may be possible to use the safety of pacemaker back-up in order to escalate beta blocker therapy for heart rate reduction.

With the focus on device programming, optimisation of CRT delivery can be considered to consist of two components: 1. Ensuring adequate biventricular pacing and 2. Optimising timing of chamber stimulation.

CRT Optimisation- Ensure Biventricular Pacing

CRT cannot be effective unless there is adequate delivery of biventricular pacing. As discussed above, to obtain this it is necessary to program carefully the upper and lower tracking rates, as well as the atrio-ventricular (AV) pacing delay. Needless to say, appropriate lead function is also essential, in particular the atrial sensitivity threshold and LV lead pacing output.

When a CRT device is interrogated, it will reveal a collection of statistics which are essential in determining whether there is adequate pacing. The heart rate histograms are obtained by continual device telemetry, recording the proportion of sensed and paced atrial and ventricular beats at different heart rates. Ventricular pacing rates of <90% require an explanation and modification. Where this is due to sinus tachycardia, an increase in the upper tracking rate may be appropriate. However, clinical judgement is required as increasing ventricular rate can compromise diastolic filling and cause a paradoxical decrease in cardiac function; in these circumstances then a pharmacological approach to heart rate reduction with beta blockers may be beneficial.

In addition, heart rate histograms may demonstrate chronotropic incompetence of the intrinsic atrial rate, in which case rate response algorithms are indicated.

Special Consideration: Dynamic AV Delay

CRT devices should normally be programmed to activate algorithms which shorten the AV pacing delay (AV delay rate response) as the heart rate increases, or when an intrinsic ventricular beat is detected (Negative AV histeresis). This helps to compensate for physiological increases in intrinsic AV node conduction during exertion.

Special Consideration: Atrial Fibrillation (and Other Atrial Arrhythmias)

Atrial tachyarrhythmias are common in patients with heart failure, and are a major cause for inadequate delivery of CRT. When high atrial rates are detected, the device will typically mode-switch into an asynchronous ventricular paced mode; where this pacing rate is below the intrinsic ventricular rate then biventricular pacing will usually cease. Aggressive control of the ventricular rate is required in patients with AF; this is often very difficult to achieve and clinical studies demonstrate poor outcomes with pharmacotherapy alone. AV node ablation has emerged as an effective treatment for persistent atrial arrhythmias in patients undergoing CRT; by electrically disconnecting the atria from the ventricles then 100% biventricular pacing is ensured. Recent studies suggest that, with this approach, outcomes in AF are improved towards the response rates seen in sinus rhythm [2].

Special Consideration: Frequent Premature Ventricular Complexes (PVCs)

Frequent PVCs are also common in heart failure. Under normal circumstances, sensed PVC will inhibit a device from delivering a biventricular pacing stimulus. Certain devices can be programmed with a ventricular-sense-pace response, such that an intrinsic beat detected in the RV will instantly trigger a pacing stimulus via the LV lead. Whilst this may allow synchronous activation where the ectopic beats originate close to the RV lead position, it is uncertain whether this programming has any real effect in reducing their impact. It may be appropriate to suppress PVCs with drug therapy, or in some cases RF ablation procedures.

CRT Optimisation- Stimulation Timing

The above measures should be undertaken to ensure that a biventricular pacing stimulus is delivered for >90% of heart beats. The second aspect of optimisation requires consideration of the timing of pacing stimuli, to ensure appropriate pacing of the ventricles with respect to the atria and each other (i.e. AV and ventriculoventricular optimiation). Post-CRT implant, usually the practice of most operators is to set the AV delay to 100-120 ms this has been deemed to satisfactory outcomes [1]. The Smart AV delay trial compared the outcomes of this approach versus echo-guided and device algorithm-based approaches and did not show significant differences in outcomes [3].

AV Optimisation

The optimal timing of the ventricular stimulation pulses relative to atrial contraction depends on a balance of two factors; intrinsic electrical conduction and diastolic ventricular filling. If the AV interval is too long, the patient's intrinsic QRS complexes may 'break through' and thwart resynchronisation. However, an interval that is too short will result in ventricular stimulation prior to the end of diastole, causing early mitral valve closure and reducing haemodynamic efficiency.

The balance between these two factors varies between patients, and there is at present no consensus as to which patients require optimisation studies, and which techniques should be utilised.

ECG Optimisation of AV Interval

In the absence of AV node disease, it might be expected that the 'physiological' AV interval should provide optimal ventricular filling, and that ventricular pacing should be timed to synchronise with the normal right ventricular activation. In its simplest form, this can be identified by the presence of fusion beats on the 12 lead ECG; invasive pressure-loop studies indicate that an optimal haemodynamic response can be obtained when left ventricular pacing spikes coincide with right bundle activation. However, as physiological AV node conduction is affected by multiple factors including autonomic state, the presence of fusion complexes may not result in reliable resynchronisation, as slight shortening of the intrinsic PR interval would result in loss of synchrony. Although the use of fusion complexes to guide programming may have an application in certain patients, it is not presently recommended routinely.

Invasive Haemodynamic Optimisation of AV Interval

Cardiac catheterisation allows the calculation of cardiac output and ventricular pressure-volume loops. Adjustment of the AV interval to maximise either cardiac output or dP/dt_{max} at the time of implant has been suggested but is not routinely performed.

Echocardiographic Optimisation of AV Interval

The American Society of Echocardiography recommendation is for consideration of echo-guided optimisation of AV interval only if the post-implant mitral inflow pattern is suggestive of stage 2 or 3 diastolic dysfunction [4]. At present, echocardiographic techniques to optimise the AV interval are the most commonly utilised.

Diastolic function (fig 1) can be assessed by examination of the E and A wave on transmitral Doppler. With an AV interval that is too short, the mitral valve closes prior to completion of diastolic filling, leading to a truncated A wave. Conversely, too long an interval causes inefficient filling with fusion of the E and A waves.

The *Iterative Method* [5] is the most commonly used echocardiographic technique to assess diastolic filling. Progressive shortening of the paced AV interval is programmed, causing separation of the E and A waves. When the A wave becomes truncated; a slight increase in the interval is then considered optimal. The best Diastolic Filling Time (DFT) calculated using the mitral valve pulse wave Doppler is deemed to proved the optimal AV delay [4]. The iterative DFT method is the most commonly used in clinical practice [6] and was also employed in the CARE-HF trial [5].

The *Ritter Method* [7] was established for the calculation of optimal AV interval for conventional pacing devices, by measuring the time between QRS onset and mitral valve closure at short and long paced intervals. This method was employed to optimise AV delay in multiple trials (MUSTIC, MIRACLE, MIRACLE –ICD) and Neither of these methods allows for direct assessment of forward systolic flow. *Aortic Outflow Methods* (fig 2) measure the velocity-time integral (VTI) of blood flow in the LV outflow tract using continuous or pulsed width Doppler. Used as a surrogate marker for stroke volume, the AV delay is adjusted until this value is maximised [8]. Similarly, in the presence of *Mitral Regurgitation*, the left ventricular pressure-volume relationship (LV dT/dt_{max}) can be estimated from the continuous wave Doppler signal of the regurgitant jet, with the AV delay adjusted to maximise this value [9]. However, these measures are highly operator-dependent as they are sensitive to the echocardiographic view and Doppler signal angle.

DEVICE-BASED OPTIMISATION OF AV INTERVAL

Recent generations of CRT devices have included a variety of algorithms that aim to identify and program an optimal AV delay based on dynamic changes to the lead electrogram. Examples include *Smart Delay (Boston Scientific)* [10] which detects intrinsic RV activation time and attempts to generate a fused LV beat, and *QuickOpt (St Jude Medical)* [11] which monitors the duration of atrial depolarisation time as a measure of diastolic filling. The SMART-AV study was a double-blinded, multi-centre study that randomised 950 patients to fixed AV-delay (120ms), echo-based optimisation or Smart-Delay based AV delay optimisation and found no difference in the primary end-point of LVESV at 6 months between the three approaches [3]. Similarly the FREEDOM study which randomised 1647 patients to either AV,VV delay optimisation using the Quick Opt algorithm or that left at operator discretion, also did not find a difference in heart failure clinical composite score [12].

Clinical Application of AV Interval Optimisation

The optimal techniques and clinical effects of AV interval optimisation remain far from convincing. However, clinical registries of CRT non-responders highlight an inappropriate AV interval as a key factor, and it appears that some individuals may improve following optimisation. In addition, acute echocardiographic and haemodynamic studies clearly demonstrate reversible improvements in cardiac output during AV interval optimisation. It is possible that optimising AV delay during exercise could lead to more consistent prediction of improved outcomes [6].

Ventriculo-Ventriculo (V-V) Optimisation

In principle, optimisation of the relative timings of left and right ventricles should result in improved mechanical function. For example, in the presence of large scars on the posterior wall, a significant delay in LV activation might be ameliorated by programming the V-V delay to allow earlier stimulation of the LV electrode. Conversely, an inferior scar may cause delayed RV activation, and early RV stimulation may be expected to have a beneficial effect. As with AV interval optimisation, despite evidence of benefit in acute haemodynamic studies, randomised clinical studies have failed to demonstrate any significant benefit of V-V optimisation in clinical populations and its role remains controversial [13].

'Too Long' and 'Too Short' AV Delay; effect on diastolic filling

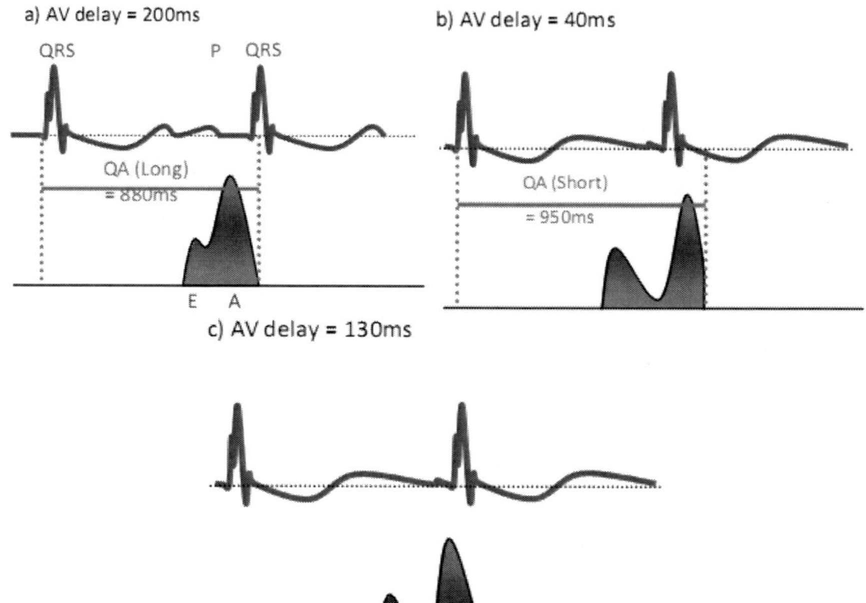

Using transmitral pulsed wave Doppler, the timing of diastolic filling is identified relative to the beginning of the QRS complex on the surface ECG.

With a long AV delay (a), the E and A waves are superimposed and diastolic filling is largely complete prior to ventricular depolarisation. With a short AV delay (b), the E and A waves are widely separated; the A wave is truncated by early closure of the mitral valve.

Using Ritter's formula, the optimal AV delay is calculated by $AV_{Short} + ([AV_{Long} + QA_{Long}] - [AV_{Short} + QA_{Short}]) = 40 + ([200 + 880] - [40 + 950]) = 130ms$

At the optimal AV interval (c), the E and A waves are clearly defined with no evidence of A wave truncation.

The principles of V-V optimisation are similar to those of A-V optimisation, with echocardiographic measurements of diastolic function, mitral valve closure and aortic outflow being the most widely used. In addition, advanced echocardiographic techniques including tissue Doppler imaging can allow an assessment of individual ventricular segments to quantify the overall degree of dyssynchrony at different V-V intervals. Such techniques are time-consuming and, as yet, not validated in clinical studies.

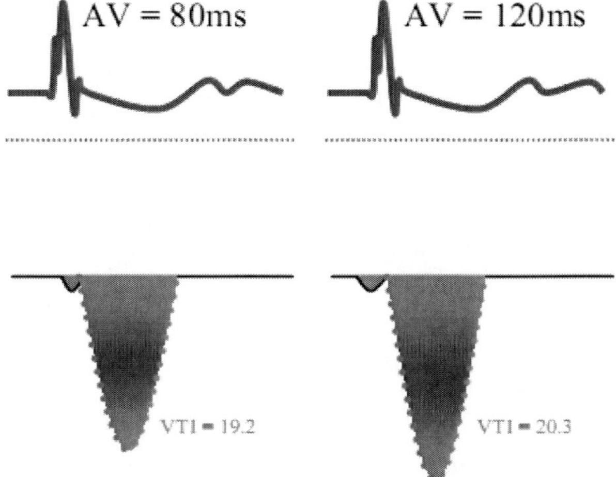

LVOT VTI Method for AV Optimisation.
Using pulse wave Doppler in the LV outflow tract, the systolic waveform is traced to give a velocity-time integral (VTI). This is a surrogate measure of cardiac output, and the AV delay can be adjusted to maximise its value.

REFERENCES

[1] Daubert JC, Saxon L, Adamson PB, et al. 2012 EHRA/HRS expert consensus statement on cardiac resynchronization therapy in heart failure: implant and follow-up recommendations and management. *Heart Rhythm.* 2012 Sep;9(9):1524-76.

[2] Ganesan AN, Brooks AG, Roberts-Thomson KC, et al. Role of AV nodal ablation in cardiac resynchronization in patients with coexistent atrial fibrillation and heart failure a systematic review. *J. Am. Coll. Cardiol.* 2012 Feb 21;59(8):719-26.

[3] Ellenbogen KA, Gold MR, Meyer TE, et al. Primary results from the SmartDelay determined AV optimization: a comparison to other AV delay methods used in cardiac resynchronization therapy (SMART-AV) trial: a randomized trial comparing empirical, echocardiography-guided, and algorithmic atrioventricular delay programming in cardiac resynchronization therapy. *Circulation* 2010 Dec 21;122(25):2660-8.

[4] Gorcsan J, III, Abraham T, Agler DA, et al. Echocardiography for cardiac resynchronization therapy: recommendations for performance and reporting--a report from the American Society of Echocardiography

Dyssynchrony Writing Group endorsed by the Heart Rhythm Society. *J. Am. Soc. Echocardiogr* 2008 Mar;21(3):191-213.

[5] Cleland JG, Daubert JC, Erdmann E, et al. The effect of cardiac resynchronization on morbidity and mortality in heart failure. *N. Engl. J. Med.* 2005 Apr 14;352(15):1539-49.

[6] Antonini L, Auriti A, Pasceri V, et al. Optimization of the atrioventricular delay in sequential and biventricular pacing: physiological bases, critical review, and new purposes. *Europace* 2012 Jul;14(7):929-38.

[7] Ritter P, Dib JC, Lelievre T. Quick determination of the optimal AV delay at rest in patients paced in DDD mode for complete AV block [abstract]. *Eur. J. CPE* 1994;4(2).

[8] Vanderheyden M, De BT, Rivero-Ayerza M, et al. Tailored echocardiographic interventricular delay programming further optimizes left ventricular performance after cardiac resynchronization therapy. *Heart Rhythm* 2005 Oct;2(10):1066-72.

[9] Morales MA, Startari U, Panchetti L, et al. Atrioventricular delay optimization by doppler-derived left ventricular dP/dt improves 6-month outcome of resynchronized patients. *Pacing Clin. Electrophysiol.* 2006 Jun;29(6):564-8.

[10] Gold MR, Niazi I, Giudici M, et al. A prospective comparison of AV delay programming methods for hemodynamic optimization during cardiac resynchronization therapy. *J. Cardiovasc. Electrophysiol.* 2007 May;18(5):490-6.

[11] Baker JH, McKenzie J, III, Beau S, et al. Acute evaluation of programmer-guided AV/PV and VV delay optimization comparing an IEGM method and echocardiogram for cardiac resynchronization therapy in heart failure patients and dual-chamber ICD implants. *J. Cardiovasc Electrophysiol.* 2007 Feb;18(2):185-91.

[12] Abraham WT, Gras D, Yu CM, et al. Rationale and design of a randomized clinical trial to assess the safety and efficacy of frequent optimization of cardiac resynchronization therapy: the Frequent Optimization Study Using the QuickOpt Method (FREEDOM) trial. *Am. Heart J.* 2010 Jun;159(6):944-8.

[13] Boriani G, Muller CP, Seidl KH, et al. Randomized comparison of simultaneous biventricular stimulation versus optimized interventricular delay in cardiac resynchronization therapy. The Resynchronization for the HemodYnamic Treatment for Heart Failure Management II

implantable cardioverter defibrillator (RHYTHM II ICD) study. *Am. Heart J.* 2006 May;151(5):1050-8.

Chapter 6

NON-RESPONDERS

INTRODUCTION: THE CHALLENGE FACING CRT

Cardiac resynchronisation therapy (CRT) has been shown to improve quality of life, NYHA class and exercise capacity [3, 4, 5], improve ejection fraction, reduce severity of mitral regurgitation, and cause reverse remodelling of the left ventricle [5], reduce hospitalisations from HF, and prolong survival [6]. Its use has accordingly been incorporated into ESC and ACC/AHA/HRS guidelines and is firmly established in the therapeutic strategy for CHF.

Yet despite its success, CRT has been hampered by the fact that a significant proportion of patients, in the region of up to 30% and possibly even more, fail to show any apparent clinical benefit from having the device, the so called "non-responders" [7, 8, 9]. In addition there is a lack of reverse remodelling in up to half of CRT patients [10]. Although there has been much research and interest in this area and better understanding as to why these patients fail to respond, the problem is not any closer to being resolved.

With an increasing CHF population, expansion in the indications for CRT in the latest guidelines [2, 11] and thus increasing number of patients eligible for CRT implantation, the number of non-responders to CRT is likely to rise. CRT is an expensive and labour- consuming procedure, associated with procedural risks to the patient, and a lifetime committed to regular follow up, device revisions and generator changes, the problem of non-response poses a very real and significant challenge to the progress of CRT, affecting both the patient and the physician, and having a huge impact on healthcare resources and cardiology services. However the issue of non-response is complex as it is multi-factorial. The definition of satisfactory response itself is controversial.

Further, similar to any therapy expectation of 100% efficacy is far from realistic. Besides these points, patients also may not respond to CRT because they were wrongly selected for CRT implant in the first place. Improvement in CRT efficacy therefore requires a multi-pronged approach. This chapter aims to highlight the main issues surrounding non-response and offer a practical approach to the cardiologist assessing and managing the non-responder.

Assessing Non-Response: Inherent Problems

Defining Non-Response

One of the main problems concerning response to CRT is that our definition (that of classifying patients into "responders" and "non–responders") - is possibly too simplistic. "Clinical non-response" has been defined as lack of improvement in symptoms of breathlessness or NYHA class/CCS class at six months and has been identified in up to 30% CRT recipients [12, 13]. "Echocardiographic non-response" (15% decrease in LV end-systolic volume) can be identified in up to 45% of CRT patients [12, 13]. "Super-responders" show a ≥30% reduction in LVESV or demonstrate the highest quartile of LVEF increase [13, 14].

In reality, patients with CHF do not neatly fall into one category or another. There is a spectrum of response, with some patients experiencing clinical deterioration, others noticing no change in their condition, and groups responding in varying degrees from mild, moderate to significant improvement in their condition [7, 8, 9].

HF has been shown to be a progressive disorder with appearance of ventricular remodelling that can precede onset of symptoms even by years and also persist and worsen despite treatment [15]. Thus, achieving haemodynamic stability in patients, despite lack of change in symptoms or echocardiographic parameters, can still be considered as a success, as the device has prevented deterioration in their clinical condition [16].

It has been shown that even though patients may not feel any better, turning the device off makes them feel considerably worse [16]. This therefore cannot be considered a failure of therapy. Conversely, in some cases, patients may feel less breathless, with no objective change in measured endpoints, which may simply be a placebo effect [17] and therefore end up being classified as responders.

Timing of Assessment of Response

Another problem is that CHF itself is difficult to predict, following a fluctuating course consisting of periods of decompensation followed by varying periods of clinical stability where patients remain haemodynamically stable with little change in symptoms. Disease progression can be heterogeneous among different patients and even in the same patient at various moments [8]. Classifying a response to CRT may vary according to the stage of the disease at which response is assessed. For example if you assess the patient six months post CRT implant (as many previous studies have done) and they are at that moment undergoing a period of CHF decompensation triggered by an infection or arrhythmia, they may be classified as a non-responder but if that same patient is assessed a year later after the triggering event has been treated and things have settled they may be now classified a responder.

Endpoints Used to Define Response

Endpoints used to assess CRT response also vary between various studies - from NYHA functional class, six minute walk test, maximal oxygen uptake on cardiopulmonary exercise testing, quality of life as assessed by the Minnesota Living with Heart Failure Questionnaire, to echocardiographic parameters such as LVEF, severity of mitral regurgitation, LV end diastolic and systolic diameters and measures of ventricular dyssynchrony, to CHF hospitalisations and mortality. It is well known that there is poor correlation between indicators of cardiac contractility and symptomatic status or exercise capacity [15]. For instance, patients with very low EF could be asymptomatic whereas patients with mild LV impairment could exhibit rest symptoms. Therefore what is classified as a good or bad response depends on what outcome or parameter is being assessed. Some parameters, such as assessing the functional status of a patient as a response, can also be quite subjective and be very much dependent on the patient's education and expectation as to what they feel CRT can provide for them [8, 17]. Several non-cardiac factors (lung function, neuro-hormonal and autonomic activity, peripheral vascular function as well as musculoskeletal factors) could add to exercise incapacity [15]. Thus CRT could lead to haemodynamic improvement without any improvement in symptoms or exercise capacity due to persisting non-cardiac factors or symptomatic improvement may be delayed by even several months. A heart failure patient with coexistent chronic obstructive airway disease (COAD), may have improved their ejection fraction significantly, and live longer as a result of their CRT device but may still feel short of breath due to their COAD and feel that they are no better with the device in. Other endpoints may be harder and more objective but may not be relevant to what the patient wants. A response therefore can also be defined as to what the patient expects and wants from the treatment – someone in NYHA class IV who is very symptomatic may simply want to be less breathless and have a better quality of life, whereas someone whose symptoms are stable may be more interested on CRT in prolonging their survival [8].

In summary, these issues illustrate the difficulties in assessing and defining non-response to CRT, with there being no clear consensus or guidelines yet offering a standardised method. From the patient's perspective the main factors that are likely to concern them are symptoms, mainly being breathless, being free from hospitalisations, and longevity of life. The physician therefore has to, taking into account a variety of factors, tailor his or her approach to the individual patient they have before them and provide them with appropriate information and educate them accordingly so they know what to expect. Although guidelines tell us who meet criteria for CRT, they do not tell us who will respond to therapy or how well they will respond. Are there any tools we can use to predict the degree of response and non-response? This shall be the focus of the next section.

Predictors of Poor Response

- *QRS duration<150msec:* The earlier studies of Pacing Therapies in Congestive Heart Failure (PATH-CHF I and II) demonstrated the role of baseline QRS duration as key determinant of response to CRT [4, 18, 19]. In particular, significant improvements in exercise capacity, peak oxygen consumption and quality of life in patients with moderate to severe heart failure were mainly seen among patients with a QRS duration > 150ms [4], whilst at QRS durations between 120ms and 150ms CRT was less efficacious at improving these parameters [8, 19]. Other studies have also showed that responders had longer initial QRS duration and greater mean QRS shortening post CRT, whilst unchanged or prolonged QRS duration after CRT was associated with higher mortality [20, 21]. Unpaced QRS duration of 120-140 msec predicted worse outcome in event-driven end-points such as echocardiographic parameters, hospitalisations and mortality [6, 22, 23, 24, 25, 26]. Sipahi et al combined 5 studies of CRT with around 6000 patients of all NYHA classes in a recent meta-analysis and showed that clinical benefit from CRT is limited to patients with QRS duration ≥ 150 msec [27]. There was a significant reduction in composite clinical end-points such as deaths and hospitalisations only amongst patients with QRS duration>150 msec (RR 0.60; 95% CI 0.53-0.67, P<0.001) in contrast to the lack of benefit amongst patients with QRS duration 120-149 msec (RR 0.95; 95% CI 0.92-1.10, P=0.49). QRS duration has hence been incorporated as the major criterion in guidelines for CRT [1, 2]. However nearly 10% of CRT patients in the "real-world" have been shown to have a base-line QRS duration of ≤130msec [28].

- *Non-LBBB QRS morphologies:* More recently, Sweeney et al demonstrated that typical LBBB was a strong predictor of response to CRT [29]. The MADIT-CRT, CARE-HF and RAFT studies demonstrated the highest response rate where dyssynchrony is due to LBBB [6, 25], and suggest that patients with RBBB respond poorly to CRT. Other analyses have also shown a lack of evidence for benefit from CRT in patients with non-LBBB QRS morphologies [30, 31, 32]. A meta-analysis of over 5300 patients from four randomised controlled trials showed that there was a significant reduction in clinical events such as all-cause mortality and CHF hospitalisations only amongst patients with LBBB QRS morphology (RR0.64; 95% CI 0.52-0.77, P<0.001) in comparison to the lack of significant benefit in patients with non-LBBB QRS morphologies (RR 0.97 ;95% CI 0.82-1.15, p0.75)[33]. This was particularly so amongst patients with RBBB (RR 0.91; 95% CI 0.69-1.2, P=0.49) or non-specific intra-ventricular conduction delay (RR1.19; 95% CI 0.87-1.63, P=0.28). However there is some evidence from other studies showing benefit in patients with advanced heart failure and non-LBBB QRS morphologies only if associated with severe QRS prolongation (i.e, >150 ms) [23, 34]. There is thus consensus between both American as well as European guidelines which strongly recommend (Class 1 indication) CRT only where the widened QRS is of a LBBB morphology and non-LBBB morphologies have received weaker recommendations.
- *Ischaemic aetiology of HF and scar burden:* Patients with non-ischaemic cardiomyopathy have been shown to respond better than

those with ischaemic aetiology [1, 2, 35]. Thus the scar burden in ischaemic cardiomyopathy has been shown to be a significant predictor of non-response to CRT [36, 37].

- *Non-ambulatory NYHA Class symptoms and severe non-cardiac co-morbidities*: Patients with refractory /non-ambulatory NYHA Class 4 symptoms, including those with end-stage HF or on inotropes respond poorly to CRT [1]. Majority of the early CRT trials enrolled patients with NYHA Class 3 status and relatively few patients (approximately 10% with NYHA Class 4 symptoms were enrolled [2]. The COMPANION study included around 200 patients with stable class IV symptoms. It should be noted that these patients were stable without unscheduled hospital admissions in the month prior to study entry, and with an expected survival of at least 6 months. CRT was associated with an improved functional performance and symptom score; however, although mortality was modestly reduced it remained very high even with therapy (2 year mortality 45% vs 62% in controls). Patients with severe non-cardiac co-morbidities (such as severe lung disease, end-stage renal failure, severe pulmonary hypertension, morbid obesity) have also shown poor response to CRT in small studies as these patients were excluded from the landmark CRT trials [1].
- *Response prediction scores*: Using multiple parameters, a response-prediction score by Moss et al, has been shown to predict echocardiographic response at 1 year [25]. Seven parameters were shown to predict response (female gender, non-ischaemic aetiology, LBBB, QRS duration≥150 ms, previous hospitalisation for heart failure, LVEDV≥125ml/m^2, left atrial volume<40 ml/m^2). Every added point from this score has shown a 13% increase in clinical benefit from CRTD. There is significant overlap of most of these parameters with the six factors which were shown to predict "super-responders" in the MADIT-CRT Trial (female sex, no previous MI, QRS≥150ms, LBBB, body mass index< 30 kg/m^2 and smaller left atrial volume index) [14].

USE OF IMAGING TO PREDICT RESPONSE

One of the main problems with QRS duration, though, is that it is simply a surrogate marker for dyssynchrony. It is well known that electrical dyssynchrony (as seen on surface ECG as LBBB with QRS > 120ms) does not always correlate with mechanical dyssynchrony (as seen on echocardiography), which in itself is a complex phenomenon, occurring at inter-ventricular, intra-ventricular and intra-mural levels [38, 39]. There were therefore many studies looking at whether echocardiographic measures could predict outcome. Yu et al [40] demonstrated that reduction in left ventricular (LV) end-systolic volume (ESV) of at least 10% after CRT resulted in excellent outcome, with patients showing significant reverse remodelling and survival rate of 90% at 3 years follow up. Similarly, Ypenburg et al [41] showed that both hospitalization and mortality correlated to the amount of change in LVESV, with patients who showed further dilatation of LVESV having the highest event rate (70% at 3 year follow up) whilst patients how showed near normalisation of LVESV only had 6% event rate. Many other studies similarly suggested that echocardiographic parameters and assessment of dyssynchrony with tissue Doppler imaging (TDI) was the way forward in predicting response to CRT [42, 43, 44, 45, 46].

All these studies paved the way for the PROSPECT (Predictors of Response to CRT) Trial [10, 13], a large, prospective, multicenter trial which assessed 498 patients with standard CRT indications (NYHA III/IV heart failure, EF < 35%, QRS > 130ms, stable medical therapy) against twelve echocardiographic parameters of dyssynchrony, based on conventional and tissue Doppler methods, to assess if any of these parameters to accurately predict positive CRT response.

The results of the trial showed that no single echocardiographic measure of ventricular dyssynchrony was able to accurately distinguish responders from non-responders in a way that would affect clinical decision making, due to intra-observer variation and large variations in sensitivity and specificity. Similarly the REthinQ (Cardiac Resynchronization Therapy in Heart Failure with Narrow QRS Complexes) trial [47] assessed the use of CRT in heart failure patients with standard CRT indications but with narrow QRS complexes and echocardiographic measures of dyssynchrony, evaluating against the primary endpoint of peak oxygen consumption on cardiopulmonary exercise testing at six months. Again the results showed that CRT did not improve peak oxygen consumption in patients with moderate to severe heart failure with narrow QRS complexes, providing evidence that patients with heart failure and narrow QRS durations may not benefit from CRT, and that echocardiographic measures of dyssynchrony were not sufficient to predict response [46]. The results of PROSPECT and REthinQ dealt a heavy blow to the use of echocardiographic measures in trying to assess CRT response, and therefore these still are not incorporated in any guidelines whilst QRS duration, a measure of electrical dyssynchrony (although not perfect) continues to remain a mainstay in CRT indications. The amount of scar ("scar burden") present has also been shown to be associated with a poor response to CRT, particularly if trans-mural and in the postero-lateral region [36, 37] (a common position for the LV lead). This has also been demonstrated in myocardial perfusion studies [37, 48], and more recently with the use of cardiac magnetic resonance imaging (CMR) [49, 50]. This approach could particularly be useful whilst evaluating patients with previous MI but the applicability of scar imaging to select ideal candidates for CRT in the "real world" remains limited at the moment due to cost and resource implications.

ROLE OF SERUM BIOMARKERS

Other studies have looked at biomarkers as predictors of CRT response such as plasma N-terminal pro B-type natriuretic peptide [51] (NT-proBNP), carboxy-terminal propeptide of procollagen type I (a marker of myocardial fibrosis) [52], and even expression of myocardial genes that regulate contractile function and pathologic hypertrophy [53]. These have all been encouraging, particularly NT-proBNP. The percentage drop of NT-proBNP post CRT was a statistically significant predictor of long term clinical improvement at three months follow up [51]. Serum bio-markers can thus have a role in assessing CRT response.

Table 1. Summary of parameters associated with CRT response can be seen in Table 1 below (# - data from large, prospective, multicenter randomised trials; *- data from smaller studies)

	Likely Response to CRT	
	Better	Worse
Predictors		
Gender #	Female	Male
Aetiology #	DCM	IHD
QRS duration #	>150ms	<120ms
QRS morphology #	Typical LBBB	RBBB, IVCD
Septal rebound stretch[54]*	Present	Absent
Posterolateral scar*	Absent	Present
Prior Dyssynchrony*	Present	Absent
% NT-proBNP drop*	High	Low

CRT trials have used several other subjective and objective parameters to measure response. These include functional assessments such as 6 minute walk test and peak VO_2 assessment on cardiopulmonary exercise testing. Of these the 6 minute walk test is a simple inexepensive functional test that can be conducted pre-implant and then three to six months post-implant to assess change in functional status [1]. The Minnesota Living with Heart Failure questionnaire can be used to assess change in quality of life due to CRT [1].

AN APPROACH TO THE NON-RESPONDER: ASSESSING THE PATIENT

When faced with the patient who fails to respond to CRT, a thorough assessment should be made to establish the cause. The first step should be to take a focussed history and perform a clinical examination. The following points should be considered:

1. *Address lifestyle factors*: Is the patient compliant with heart failure medications? Is there room for further up-titration of ACE inhibitors and B-blockers? Do their diuretics need to be increased or other medications added? Are they aware of salt and fluid restrictions? Are they appropriately educated about their condition? What are their expectations? Has smoking cessation been addressed? Is weight an issue? Are they getting adequate exercise/cardiac rehabilitation?
2. *Address non-cardiac medical problems:* The cardiologist needs to ensure that symptoms are mainly due to their heart failure, before labelling this as non-response to CRT. Often patient's symptoms are multi-factorial with other medical problems confounding the issue (such as chronic obstructive airway disease, anaemia, chest infections leading to CHF decompensation, worsening renal function etc.) d with heart failure) or do they have worsening renal failure? Further investigation with full set of blood tests, including FBC, U+E and CRP, and a chest X-ray may be helpful.
3. *Look for arrhythmias:* There is a strong association between heart failure and atrial fibrillation (AF), a fact that is underrepresented in the literature with most studies and trials being performed in patients in sinus rhythm [55]. When AF is present in heart failure patients it is associated with higher morbidity and mortality [56]. It is also more

likely the more severe the heart failure, being present in anywhere from 30-50% of heart failure patients [57]. If AF or flutter is found to be present it can interfere with biventricular (BiV) pacing, preventing the target of 90% BiV pacing from being achieved, resulting in impaired clinical response. In this case, up-titrate B-blockers to achieve higher grade block at the AV node, and refer for consideration of AV nodal ablation. There is emerging body of evidence that AV node ablation to achieve maximum BiV pacing confers significant clinical benefit in this group of patients [58, 59]. Another frequent finding is frequent PVCs that can interfere with BiV Pacing – if this is the case, again B-blockers can be increased, ensure the device has PVC response switched on, and in rare cases ablation may be considered. If episodes of ventricular tachycardia are noted, consider upgrading device from CRT-P to CRT-D and if VT episodes are very frequent, consider VT ablation.

4. *Assess coronary arteries and cardiac structures*: If there is a history of IHD, consider performing a functional assessment with either myocardial perfusion scanning or dobutamine stress echocardiography to look for viability and stress inducible ischaemia. This can detect if there is myocardium that can be salvaged by coronary artery revascularisation. Equally if not performed recently, a repeat echocardiogram will help evaluate cardiac structures and provide valuable information. Is there a pericardial effusion? Does this need draining? What does LV function look like now post CRT implant? It will also help assess if there is any significant valvular disease contributing to symptoms, such as progression of underlying aortic stenosis or if there is any severe MR present. If there is, would this patient be a candidate for transcutaneous aortic valve implantation (TAVI) or mitral clip insertion?

Once all factors pertaining to the patient have been examined, the next step would be to assess the CRT pacing system itself.

Issues with Lead Positioning

Assessment of LV lead position is crucial and is a significant cause of non-response to CRT [17, 60, 61]. To achieve maximum resynchronisation and hence best clinical response the LV lead needs to be placed in a lateral, or posterolateral cardiac vein. This is because LV free wall sites are usually the latest to be activated and stimulating these sites reliably restores homogenous LV activation, significantly improving dyssynchrony. Conversely, anterior wall regions are usually activated early, and pacing these sites can enhance regional dyssynchrony and worsen LV function, causing clinical deterioration [17]. Similarly apical pacing sites have also led to poor outcomes [62]. However, these features are not universally observed due to heterogeneity in the activation pattern such that the anterior wall could also be the segment with most delayed activation in LBBB and heart failure [63, 64].

Various factors can cause sub-optimal LV lead positioning and function – this may be related to operator experience, variation in coronary venous anatomy, limiting access and delivery of the lead to the most suitable site of myocardium, problem of diaphragmatic twitching (due to close proximity of left phrenic nerve to lateral LV wall) limiting optimal lead positioning, and LV lead displacement occurring onto a region of infarcted, scarred myocardium or site that does not provide effective pacing. A PA and lateral chest CXR (and comparison to previous chest film) will help identify lead position, and if displaced or problematic, patient will need to have this LV lead re-positioned into more suitable branch for effective LV pacing (see figures A, B and C below). Equally if no better target veins are identified, then patient could be considered for surgical epicardial LV lead placement. More recently, there has also been interest in transseptal endocardial LV lead placement (this shall be discussed more in the next chapter).

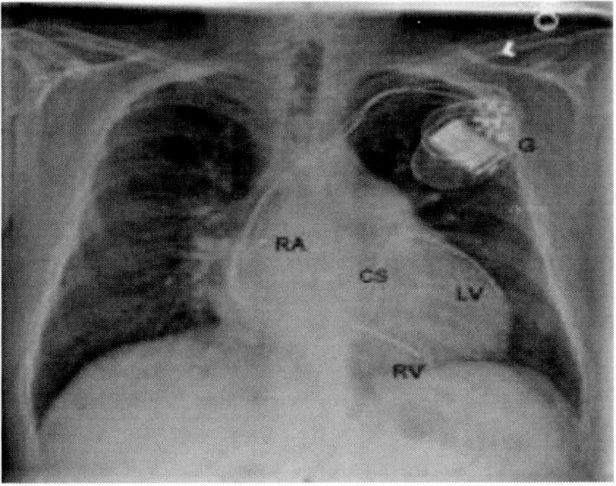

Figure A. Suitable position of LV lead in lateral vein.

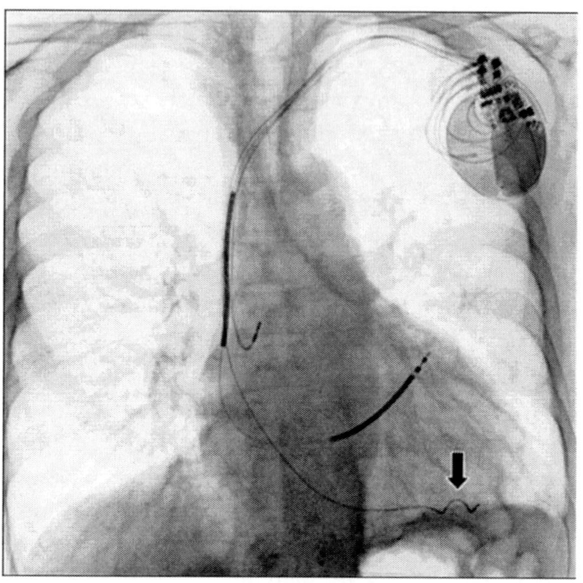

Figure B. LV lead in mid cardiac vein.

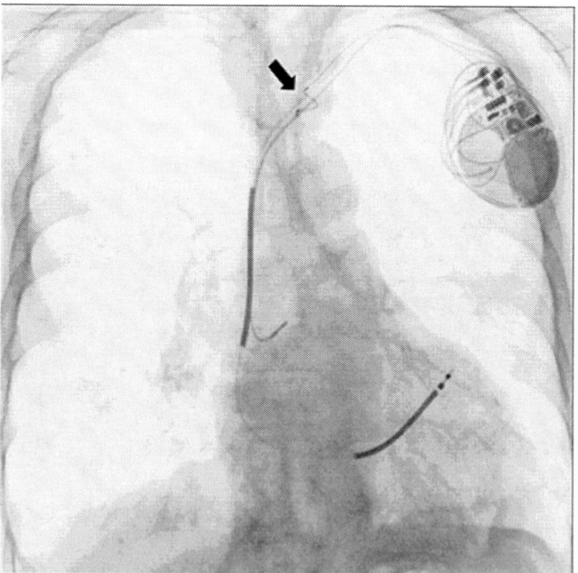

Figure C. Displaced back into inominate vein.

Aside from lead position, all usual pacing parameters such as threshold, sensitivity and impedance, should be assessed, and device and all leads checked. Alow impedance could imply insulation break, while high impedance conductor/lead fracture and this would need to be managed. Equally, rise in threshold with normal impedance could suggest LV lead displacement onto scarred myocardium, requiring re-positioning.

OPTIMISING DEVICE PROGRAMMING

In a small number of non-responders, optimising device programming by adjusting ventricle-to-ventricle (V-V) or atria-to-ventricle (A-V) timing delays in order to optimize ventricular function, may be of benefit.

Often the AV delay is programmed at a nominal low value of around 100-120ms to ensure maximum BiV pacing though this may excessively reduce atrial contribution to LV filling. Some studies suggest maintaining intrinsic AV conduction in non-responders to avoid this [65].

Similarly, output and timing of right and left ventricular stimulation can be programmed to optimise inter-ventricular delay. Whilst some patients respond well to simultaneous BiV pacing, others do better with pre-activation of the right ventricle before the left. In this respect there is considerable inter-individual variability, and fine-tuning of the V-V interval has to be tailored to the individual to gain maximum benefit.

Whilst large interventricular delays (up to 100ms) can be programmed, optimal settings for V-V delay seem to be in a relatively narrow range (12-20ms) [17]. Several methods can be used to achieve optimisation, most are echo based (*covered in detail in chapter 5*).

These include Doppler measures of mitral inflow velocity, and LV outflow velocity as markers for LV filling and ejection [60], aortic valve velocity time integral optimization, and M-mode with septal to posterior wall times.

In addition to this, electrocadiographic-based QRS duration measures and, more recently, intra-cardiac electrogram (IEG)-based optimization, can be utilized. Whilst this can be used for particular patients who fail to respond to CRT, recent literature and studies, particularly the FREEDOM [66] and the RHYTHM II ICD [67] trial, suggest that there is no difference in clinical outcome in patients having frequent AV and VV optimizations compared with routine optimization strategy.

This may mean that AV and VV optimization may play a less significant role in the management of the non-responder. Interestingly, in optimising device programming, some studies have also suggested anodal stimulation (i.e. pacing from LV lead (cathode) to RV coil or ring (anode)) that resulting in unintentional RV pacing may be an under-recognized cause of nonresponse [68], and may also have to be assessed.

Conclusion – "Non-Responder or Cannot Respond"

It is important to recognize that in a sub-set of patients their deterioration in symptoms is not due to a genuine non-response to CRT per se, but a reflection of deterioration in their underlying pathology. These patients are exhibiting an irreversible progression in their heart failure towards the advanced, end stages [60]. Rather than non-response, these patients simply "cannot respond". Despite several advancements in heart failure management over the years, its prognosis remains poor, and inevitably the cardiologist will encounter heart failure patients reaching these final stages. At this point, difficult decisions need to be made as to what further management will involve. If full active treatment is to continue, then the patient may require inotropic support, and be considered for left ventricular assist device (LVAD) as a bridge, or need working up for heart transplant. If, due to various co-morbidities, this is not an option, then management should involve end of life care, symptom control, and palliation. This should be conducted by a full multi-disciplinary team approach, with heart failure nurses, cardiologists, and cardiac transplant surgeons, with close involvement of patients and their relatives in the decision-making process.

References

[1] Daubert JC, Saxon L, Adamson PB, et al. 2012 EHRA/HRS expert consensus statement on cardiac resynchronization therapy in heart failure: implant and follow-up recommendations and management. *Heart Rhythm* 2012 Sep;9(9):1524-76.

[2] Tracy CM, Epstein AE, Darbar D, et al. 2012 ACCF/AHA/HRS Focused Update of the 2008 Guidelines for Device-Based Therapy of Cardiac

Rhythm Abnormalities: A Report of the American College of Cardiology Foundation/American Heart Association Task Force on Practice Guidelines. *Heart Rhythm* 2012 Oct;9(10):1737-53.

[3] Abraham WT, Fisher WG, Smith AL, et al. Cardiac resynchronization in chronic heart failure. *N. Engl. J. Med.* 2002 Jun 13;346(24):1845-53.

[4] Auricchio A, Stellbrink C, Butter C, et al. Clinical efficacy of cardiac resynchronization therapy using left ventricular pacing in heart failure patients stratified by severity of ventricular conduction delay. *J. Am. Coll. Cardiol.* 2003 Dec 17;42(12):2109-16.

[5] Linde C, Leclercq C, Rex S, et al. Long-term benefits of biventricular pacing in congestive heart failure: results from the MUltisite STimulation in cardiomyopathy (MUSTIC) study. *J. Am. Coll. Cardiol.* 2002 Jul 3;40(1):111-8.

[6] Cleland JG, Daubert JC, Erdmann E, et al. The effect of cardiac resynchronization on morbidity and mortality in heart failure. *N. Engl. J. Med.* 2005 Apr 14;352(15):1539-49.

[7] Zaca V, Mondillo S, Gaddi R, et al. Profiling cardiac resynchronization therapy patients: responders, non-responders and those who cannot respond--the good, the bad and the ugly? *Int. J. Cardiovasc. Imaging* 2011 Jan;27(1):51-7.

[8] Auricchio A, Prinzen FW. Non-responders to cardiac resynchronization therapy: the magnitude of the problem and the issues. *Circ. J.* 2011;75(3):521-7.

[9] Cleland JG, Tavazzi L, Daubert JC, et al. Cardiac resynchronization therapy: are modern myths preventing appropriate use? *J. Am. Coll. Cardiol.* 2009 Feb 17;53(7):608-11.

[10] Chung ES, Leon AR, Tavazzi L, et al. Results of the Predictors of Response to CRT (PROSPECT) trial. *Circulation* 2008 May 20;117(20):2608-16.

[11] McMurray JJ, Adamopoulos S, Anker SD, et al. ESC Guidelines for the diagnosis and treatment of acute and chronic heart failure 2012: The Task Force for the Diagnosis and Treatment of Acute and Chronic Heart Failure 2012 of the European Society of Cardiology. Developed in collaboration with the Heart Failure Association (HFA) of the ESC. *Eur. J. Heart Fail* 2012 Aug;14(8):803-69.

[12] Ypenburg C, Westenberg JJ, Bleeker GB, et al. Noninvasive imaging in cardiac resynchronization therapy--part 1: selection of patients. *Pacing Clin. Electrophysiol.* 2008 Nov;31(11):1475-99.

[13] van Bommel RJ, Bax JJ, Abraham WT, et al. Characteristics of heart failure patients associated with good and poor response to cardiac resynchronization therapy: a PROSPECT (Predictors of Response to CRT) sub-analysis. *Eur. Heart J.* 2009 Oct;30(20):2470-7.
[14] Hsu JC, Solomon SD, Bourgoun M, et al. Predictors of super-response to cardiac resynchronization therapy and associated improvement in clinical outcome: the MADIT-CRT (multicenter automatic defibrillator implantation trial with cardiac resynchronization therapy) study. *J. Am. Coll. Cardiol.* 2012 Jun 19;59(25):2366-73.
[15] Hunt SA, Abraham WT, Chin MH, et al. 2009 Focused update incorporated into the ACC/AHA 2005 Guidelines for the Diagnosis and Management of Heart Failure in Adults A Report of the American College of Cardiology Foundation/American Heart Association Task Force on Practice Guidelines Developed in Collaboration With the International Society for Heart and Lung Transplantation. *J. Am. Coll. Cardiol.* 2009 Apr 14;53(15):e1-e90.
[16] Mullens W, Verga T, Grimm RA, et al. Persistent hemodynamic benefits of cardiac resynchronization therapy with disease progression in advanced heart failure. *J. Am. Coll. Cardiol.* 2009 Feb 17;53(7):600-7.
[17] Fox DJ, Fitzpatrick AP, Davidson NC. Optimisation of cardiac resynchronisation therapy: addressing the problem of "non-responders". *Heart* 2005 Aug;91(8):1000-2.
[18] Auricchio A, Stellbrink C, Block M, et al. Effect of pacing chamber and atrioventricular delay on acute systolic function of paced patients with congestive heart failure. The Pacing Therapies for Congestive Heart Failure Study Group. The Guidant Congestive Heart Failure Research Group. *Circulation* 1999 Jun 15;99(23):2993-3001.
[19] Auricchio A, Stellbrink C, Sack S, et al. Long-term clinical effect of hemodynamically optimized cardiac resynchronization therapy in patients with heart failure and ventricular conduction delay. *J. Am. Coll. Cardiol.* 2002 Jun 19;39(12):2026-33.
[20] Lecoq G, Leclercq C, Leray E, et al. Clinical and electrocardiographic predictors of a positive response to cardiac resynchronization therapy in advanced heart failure. *Eur. Heart J.* 2005 Jun;26(11):1094-100.
[21] Kronborg MB, Nielsen JC, Mortensen PT. Electrocardiographic patterns and long-term clinical outcome in cardiac resynchronization therapy. *Europace* 2010 Feb;12(2):216-22.

[22] Bristow MR, Saxon LA, Boehmer J, et al. Cardiac-resynchronization therapy with or without an implantable defibrillator in advanced chronic heart failure. *N. Engl. J. Med.* 2004 May 20;350(21):2140-50.

[23] Tang AS, Wells GA, Talajic M, et al. Cardiac-resynchronization therapy for mild-to-moderate heart failure. *N. Engl. J. Med.* 2010 Dec 16;363(25):2385-95.

[24] Stellbrink C, Breithardt OA, Franke A, et al. Impact of cardiac resynchronization therapy using hemodynamically optimized pacing on left ventricular remodeling in patients with congestive heart failure and ventricular conduction disturbances. *J. Am. Coll. Cardiol.* 2001 Dec;38(7):1957-65.

[25] Moss AJ, Hall WJ, Cannom DS, et al. Cardiac-resynchronization therapy for the prevention of heart-failure events. *N. Engl. J. Med.* 2009 Oct 1;361(14):1329-38.

[26] Daubert JC, Saxon L, Adamson PB, et al. 2012 EHRA/HRS expert consensus statement on cardiac resynchronization therapy in heart failure: implant and follow-up recommendations and management: A registered branch of the European Society of Cardiology (ESC), and the Heart Rhythm Society; and in collaboration with the Heart Failure Society of America (HFSA), the American Society of Echocardiography (ASE), the American Heart Association (AHA), the European Association of Echocardiography (EAE) of the ESC and the Heart Failure Association of the ESC (HFA). * Endorsed by the governing bodies of AHA, ASE, EAE, HFSA, HFA, EHRA, and HRS. *Europace* 2012 Sep;14(9):1236-86.

[27] Sipahi I, Carrigan TP, Rowland DY, et al. Impact of QRS duration on clinical event reduction with cardiac resynchronization therapy: meta-analysis of randomized controlled trials. *Arch. Intern. Med.* 2011 Sep 12;171(16):1454-62.

[28] Mullens W, Grimm RA, Verga T, et al. Insights from a cardiac resynchronization optimization clinic as part of a heart failure disease management program. *J. Am. Coll. Cardiol.* 2009 Mar 3;53(9):765-73.

[29] Sweeney MO, van Bommel RJ, Schalij MJ, et al. Analysis of ventricular activation using surface electrocardiography to predict left ventricular reverse volumetric remodeling during cardiac resynchronization therapy. *Circulation* 2010 Feb 9;121(5):626-34.

[30] Bilchick KC, Kamath S, Dimarco JP, et al. Bundle-branch block morphology and other predictors of outcome after cardiac

resynchronization therapy in Medicare patients. *Circulation* 2010 Nov 16;122(20):2022-30.

[31] Adelstein EC, Saba S. Usefulness of baseline electrocardiographic QRS complex pattern to predict response to cardiac resynchronization. *Am. J. Cardiol.* 2009 Jan 15;103(2):238-42.

[32] Rickard J, Kumbhani DJ, Gorodeski EZ, et al. Cardiac resynchronization therapy in non-left bundle branch block morphologies. *Pacing Clin. Electrophysiol.* 2010 May;33(5):590-5.

[33] Sipahi I, Chou JC, Hyden M, et al. Effect of QRS morphology on clinical event reduction with cardiac resynchronization therapy: meta-analysis of randomized controlled trials. *Am. Heart J.* 2012 Feb;163(2):260-7.

[34] Rickard J, Bassiouny M, Cronin EM, et al. Predictors of response to cardiac resynchronization therapy in patients with a non-left bundle branch block morphology. *Am. J. Cardiol.* 2011 Dec 1;108(11):1576-80.

[35] Jessup M, Abraham WT, Casey DE, et al. 2009 focused update: ACCF/AHA Guidelines for the Diagnosis and Management of Heart Failure in Adults: a report of the American College of Cardiology Foundation/American Heart Association Task Force on Practice Guidelines: developed in collaboration with the International Society for Heart and Lung Transplantation. *Circulation* 2009 Apr 14;119(14):1977-2016.

[36] Bleeker GB, Kaandorp TA, Lamb HJ, et al. Effect of posterolateral scar tissue on clinical and echocardiographic improvement after cardiac resynchronization therapy. *Circulation* 2006 Feb 21;113(7):969-76.

[37] Ypenburg C, Schalij MJ, Bleeker GB, et al. Impact of viability and scar tissue on response to cardiac resynchronization therapy in ischaemic heart failure patients. *Eur. Heart J.* 2007 Jan;28(1):33-41.

[38] Cho GY, Kim HK, Kim YJ, et al. Electrical and mechanical dyssynchrony for prediction of cardiac events in patients with systolic heart failure. *Heart* 2010 Jul;96(13):1029-32.

[39] Auricchio A, Yu CM. Beyond the measurement of QRS complex toward mechanical dyssynchrony: cardiac resynchronisation therapy in heart failure patients with a normal QRS duration. *Heart* 2004 May;90(5):479-81.

[40] Yu CM, Bleeker GB, Fung JW, et al. Left ventricular reverse remodeling but not clinical improvement predicts long-term survival after cardiac resynchronization therapy. *Circulation* 2005 Sep 13;112(11):1580-6.

[41] Ypenburg C, van Bommel RJ, Borleffs CJ, et al. Long-term prognosis after cardiac resynchronization therapy is related to the extent of left ventricular reverse remodeling at midterm follow-up. *J. Am. Coll. Cardiol.* 2009 Feb 10;53(6):483-90.

[42] Yu CM, Zhang Q, Fung JW, et al. A novel tool to assess systolic asynchrony and identify responders of cardiac resynchronization therapy by tissue synchronization imaging. *J. Am. Coll. Cardiol.* 2005 Mar 1;45(5):677-84.

[43] Bax JJ, Bleeker GB, Marwick TH, et al. Left ventricular dyssynchrony predicts response and prognosis after cardiac resynchronization therapy. *J. Am. Coll. Cardiol.* 2004 Nov 2;44(9):1834-40.

[44] Breithardt OA, Breithardt G. Quest for the best candidate: how much imaging do we need before prescribing cardiac resynchronization therapy? *Circulation* 2006 Feb 21;113(7):926-8.

[45] Zaret BL. Cardiac imaging and cardiac resynchronization therapy: time to get in phase. *JACC Cardiovasc. Imaging* 2008 Sep;1(5):614-6.

[46] Achilli A, Sassara M, Ficili S, et al. Long-term effectiveness of cardiac resynchronization therapy in patients with refractory heart failure and "narrow" QRS. *J. Am. Coll. Cardiol.* 2003 Dec 17;42(12):2117-24.

[47] Beshai JF, Grimm RA, Nagueh SF, et al. Cardiac-resynchronization therapy in heart failure with narrow QRS complexes. *N. Engl. J. Med.* 2007 Dec 13;357(24):2461-71.

[48] Adelstein EC, Saba S. Scar burden by myocardial perfusion imaging predicts echocardiographic response to cardiac resynchronization therapy in ischemic cardiomyopathy. *Am. Heart J.* 2007 Jan;153(1):105-12.

[49] Leyva F. Cardiac resynchronization therapy guided by cardiovascular magnetic resonance. *J. Cardiovasc. Magn Reson* 2010;12:64.

[50] Taylor AJ, Elsik M, Broughton A, et al. Combined dyssynchrony and scar imaging with cardiac magnetic resonance imaging predicts clinical response and long-term prognosis following cardiac resynchronization therapy. *Europace* 2010 May;12(5):708-13.

[51] Ding LG, Hua W, Zhang S, et al. Decrease of plasma N-terminal pro beta-type natriuretic peptide as a predictor of clinical improvement after cardiac resynchronization therapy for heart failure. *Chin. Med. J. (Engl)* 2009 Mar 20;122(6):617-21.

[52] Garcia-Bolao I, Macias A, Lopez B, et al. A biomarker of myocardial fibrosis predicts long-term response to cardiac resynchronization therapy. *J. Am. Coll. Cardiol.* 2006 Jun 6;47(11):2335-7.

[53] Vanderheyden M, Mullens W, Delrue L, et al. Myocardial gene expression in heart failure patients treated with cardiac resynchronization therapy responders versus nonresponders. *J. Am. Coll Cardiol* 2008 Jan 15;51(2):129-36.

[54] Kass DA. An epidemic of dyssynchrony: but what does it mean? *J. Am. Coll Cardiol* 2008 Jan 1;51(1):12-7.

[55] Caldwell JC, Contractor H, Petkar S, et al. Atrial fibrillation is under-recognized in chronic heart failure: insights from a heart failure cohort treated with cardiac resynchronization therapy. *Europace* 2009 Oct;11(10):1295-300.

[56] Mamas MA, Caldwell JC, Chacko S, et al. A meta-analysis of the prognostic significance of atrial fibrillation in chronic heart failure. *Eur. J. Heart Fail* 2009 Jul;11(7):676-83.

[57] Gasparini M, Regoli F. Cardiac resynchronisation therapy in patients with atrial fibrillation. *Heart* 2009 Jan;95(1):83-4.

[58] Gasparini M, Auricchio A, Regoli F, et al. Four-year efficacy of cardiac resynchronization therapy on exercise tolerance and disease progression: the importance of performing atrioventricular junction ablation in patients with atrial fibrillation. *J. Am. Coll. Cardiol.* 2006 Aug 15;48(4):734-43.

[59] Ganesan AN, Brooks AG, Roberts-Thomson KC, et al. Role of AV nodal ablation in cardiac resynchronization in patients with coexistent atrial fibrillation and heart failure a systematic review. *J. Am. Coll. Cardiol.* 2012 Feb 21;59(8):719-26.

[60] Gorcsan J, III. Finding pieces of the puzzle of nonresponse to cardiac resynchronization therapy. *Circulation* 2011 Jan 4;123(1):10-2.

[61] Herre J. Keys to successful cardiac resynchronization therapy. *Am. Heart J.* 2007 Apr;153(4 Suppl):18-24.

[62] Singh JP, Klein HU, Huang DT, et al. Left ventricular lead position and clinical outcome in the multicenter automatic defibrillator implantation trial-cardiac resynchronization therapy (MADIT-CRT) trial. *Circulation* 2011 Mar 22;123(11):1159-66.

[63] Singh JP, Heist EK, Ruskin JN, et al. "Dialing-in" cardiac resynchronization therapy: overcoming constraints of the coronary venous anatomy. *J. Interv. Card Electrophysiol.* 2006 Oct;17(1):51-8.

[64] Fung JW, Yu CM, Yip G, et al. Variable left ventricular activation pattern in patients with heart failure and left bundle branch block. *Heart* 2004 Jan;90(1):17-9.

[65] Wang RX, Guo T, Hua BT, et al. Initial experiences of maintaining atrioventricular intrinsic conduction during cardiac resynchronization therapy in non-responders. *Chin. Med. J. (Engl)* 2009 Oct 20;122(20):2455-60.

[66] Abraham WT, Gras D, Yu CM, et al. Rationale and design of a randomized clinical trial to assess the safety and efficacy of frequent optimization of cardiac resynchronization therapy: the Frequent Optimization Study Using the QuickOpt Method (FREEDOM) trial. *Am. Heart J.* 2010 Jun;159(6):944-8.

[67] Boriani G, Muller CP, Seidl KH, et al. Randomized comparison of simultaneous biventricular stimulation versus optimized interventricular delay in cardiac resynchronization therapy. The Resynchronization for the HemodYnamic Treatment for Heart Failure Management II implantable cardioverter defibrillator (RHYTHM II ICD) study. *Am. Heart J.* 2006 May;151(5):1050-8.

[68] Dendy KF, Powell BD, Cha YM, et al. Anodal stimulation: an underrecognized cause of nonresponders to cardiac resynchronization therapy. *Indian Pacing Electrophysiol. J.* 2011;11(3):64-72.

Chapter 7

FUTURE DIRECTIONS

INTRODUCTION

The first pacemaker implant in a human was performed in 1958 by Ake Senning using a device designed by Rune Elmqvist under the direction of Senning. This failed after three hours. A second device was then implanted which lasted for two days.

Following these humble beginnings, pacemaker technology has certainly made astonishing progress and advanced leaps and bounds in the last few decades to where we stand now, perhaps on the cusp of another revolution. The early 1990s heralded the advent of cardiac resynchronisation therapy (CRT). Following several major groundbreaking heart failure and device therapy trials in the mid to late 1990s, CRT has now been adopted into widespread clinical use and undergone massive expansion in the number of patients being implanted with these devices. We have seen improved miniaturisation of generators, with more complex functions and monitoring capabilities, improvements in longevity of battery life, major advances in lead design and technology and more recently seen the increasing use of remote monitoring. All these advancements have helped make pacemaker insertions more safe, comfortable and convenient for both the patient and the implanting cardiologist.

There still remains the problem, though, of non-responders, which affects about 30% of patients implanted with a CRT device, which poses a major challenge to cardiologists and the device industry [1, 2]. There is also a failure to implant LV lead in up to 10% cases due to procedural difficulties related to abnormal CS anatomy [3]. Problems related to the lead itself include pacemaker system infection requiring device and lead extraction, a procedure associated with significant morbidity and mortality. In addition, there are issues relating to diaphragmatic twitching, lead displacement, conductor fracture and insulation breaks causing inadequate pacing, which necessitates further procedures, system revisions and lead re-positioning, which again increases the risk of infection. These weaknesses related to the lead pose the Achilles' heel of pacemaker technology. There has therefore been renewed interest at ways of tackling these problems to improve and perfect CRT use for patients and implanting cardiologists. These include some novel techniques to assist LV lead implant using imaging/ mapping techniques, alternative routes for LV pacing such as trans-septal or transapical endocardial LV pacing, minimally invasive techniques for epicardial lead placement and multi-site LV pacing. Leadless technology using ultrasound or magnetic field-delivered electrical energy and biological pacemakers may also herald a new revolution. We shall elucidate these novel strategies in this chapter.

New LV Lead Technology and Implant Techniques

The main difficulty with CRT implantation is that posed by the LV lead. Ideally it needs to be placed in the lateral or postero-lateral vein to achieve optimum resynchronization, though this is easier said than done. Cannulating the coronary sinus can be challenging, and the operator is often limited by coronary venous anatomy. There may not be a suitable branch to place the LV lead in, or the branch may be so tortuous, small and degenerate or stenosed that it does not allow the lead into it. Equally pacing may be hampered by the lead being in an area of posterolateral scar giving unsatisfactory thresholds, or cause troublesome diaphragmatic twitching requiring it to be placed somewhere else less suitable.

Novel Techniques to Assist LV Lead Implant

Use of electroanatomic mapping with the Ensite NavX system (St Jude Medical, Endocardial Solutions Inc., St.Paul, MN, USA) [4] has been shown to improve accuracy of LV lead placement and also lead to a reduction in fluoroscopy time. The Niobe system (Stereotaxis Inc., St. Louis, USA) is a magnetic navigation system for LV lead implant that uses two permanent magnets on either side of the fluoroscopy table to create a steerable magnetic field. The magnetic guidewire also has a small magnet at the tip and can be remotely navigated enabling precision to allow engagement of angulated target veins and also leads to reduced fluoroscopy time [5, 6, 7, 8].

Alternative Routes for LV Lead Placement

Whilst epicardial LV lead placement is well established as an alternative means of accessing the lateral wall of the left ventricle, it has the disadvantage that it involves surgery on an already frail, sick group of patients and again there is variation in long-term results of how effective epicardial lead placement is in achieving optimum resynchronization [9].

Endocardial lead implantation by means of transseptal puncture at the atrial level offers several potential advantages. It allows access to all LV regions, overcoming the limitations of coronary venous anatomy, and endocardial ventricular layers offer faster impulse propagation than epicardial layers which might result in improved haemodynamics [10]. Combined with prior imaging or mapping techniques this could allow the LV lead to be placed in the ideal area of ventricle that is not scarred, and also the latest area to be activated, offering good pacing thresholds and optimum resynchronization. Superior electrical resynchronization and haemodynamic improvement, assessed by means of + dP/dt_{max}, has been shown with endocardial LV pacing in an acute canine model compared with epicardial stimulation, which resulted in transmural dispersion of repolarisation and less effective improvement [11]. Further studies in humans have showed mixed results. Spragg et al compared the haemodynamic effects of LV endocardial pacing in patients with ischaemic cardiomyopathy [12]. In this study, LV endocardial versus epicardial pacing at transmural sites yielded equivalent dP/dt_{max} values, suggesting no differences in haemodynamics, though superior haemodynamic results were seen in patients when endocardial pacing was performed from extreme basal sites at positions adjacent to the mitral ring (>85% increase in dP/dt_{max}). In a study by Derval et al pacing at the best LV site in 35 patients with non-ischaemic cardiomyopathy was associated with twice the improvement in + dP/dt_{max} compared to CS pacing [13]. Bracke et al also showed that left ventricular endocardial pacing improves clinical efficacy in a CRT non-responder [14]. Several papers suggest that endocardial LV pacing may be a realistic consideration for the CRT non-responder with unfavourable coronary sinus anatomy as an alternative to epicardial pacing, offering better haemodynamic benefit, particularly when the LV lead in placed in the basal postero-lateral region [15, 16, 17]. There are problems however; the procedure is technically challenging, there is increased risk of thrombo-embolism due to leads in the LV cavity (and therefore requires lifelong anticoagulation), and as lead crosses the mitral valve there is risk of mitral regurgitation and endocarditis if there is pacemaker system infection [10]. To avoid this, a trans-apical approach to endocardial LV lead placement has also been described in a limited number of patients [18].

Apart from endocardial LV lead pacing there has also been interest in various types of multisite pacing to see if this might help in the issue of non-response, the theory being that placing multiple pacing leads at different sites could create multiple waves of electrical activation, further reducing dyssynchony in the case of ventricular conduction delay [19]. Following case reports and small observational studies [20, 21], it seemed that triple ventricular pacing or triangle ventricular pacing (so called "Tri V" pacing), be it whether with an extra RV or LV lead, seemed to result in larger haemodynamic improvement compared with traditional biventricular pacing [22]. This led onto the TRIP-HF (Triple Resynchronization in Paced Heart Failure Patients) study, the first randomized prospective multicenter trial comparing triple-site stimulation (2 transvenous LV leads placed on the anterior and lateral/posterolateral LV wall, and 1 RV lead) with conventional BiV pacing. The study enrolled patients with heart failure presenting with slow atrial fibrillation, and showed that compared with standard BiV pacing, triple site ventricular stimulation promoted further LV reverse remodelling as assessed by end-systolic and end-diastolic volumes and ejection fraction at three month follow up. Long term difference in clinical outcome, though, was not shown and this question remains to be answered. Whilst multisite and endocardial pacing offer a possible alternative to improve BiV pacing in CRT non-responders, there has not been enough large scale evidence yet to bring this into routine clinical practice, and how far this changes the face of future CRT remains to be assessed.

An age-old alternative to transvenous LV lead implant is the surgical epicardial LV lead implant which was first described in 1994 [23]. Whilst this approach can offer benefits such as direct visualisation of the implanting segment, lack of need for fluoroscopy or contrast or the lack of difficulties posed by atypical CS anatomy, there are also disadvantages such as need for general anaesthesia, longer post-operative recovery time and inferior long term pacing parameters leading to a 5 year lead failure rate of 15% [9]. However surgical LV lead implant techniques have also evolved to now include less invasive techniques requiring reduced procedural times such as using the lateral mini-thoracotomy technique, video assisted thoracoscopic approaches and robotically assisted procedures [24, 25].

New LV Lead Technology

Quadripolar LV Lead

The problems with CRT are primarily related to the LV lead, which can cause phrenic nerve stimulation, diaphragmatic twitch and high capture thresholds which often results in further procedures and attempts to reposition the lead. Clinically relevant phrenic nerve stimulation has been shown to occur in about 22% of patients at CRT implant or follow up with its occurrence highest in those patients where the LV lead is at the sites most associated with reverse remodelling [26, 27].

A quadripolar left ventricular lead, the St Jude Quartet model 1458Q, has been developed to help in overcoming these problems. The Quartet lead allows ten different pacing vectors allowing the cardiologist to "electronically reposition" and change the electrode configuration to help avoid phrenic nerve stimulation and optimise pacing thresholds without having to adjust lead position. This reduces the need for procedural, manual lead repositioning, which is difficult, and time consuming, with further, longer procedures being associated with higher chance of infection and need for extraction. This quadripolar lead therefore not only allows programming flexibility but also offers more options to achieve effective and safe CRT.

These findings have also been confirmed in the literature [27, 28, 29], and the Quartet lead has already started to be used in clinical practice and forms a useful tool in the cardiologist's armamentarium in enhancing CRT success, and reducing phrenic nerve stimulation. Certainly it appears likely that the Quartet will become a more widely used, and established piece of kit in CRT implantation, at least for the near future. See figures 1 and 2.

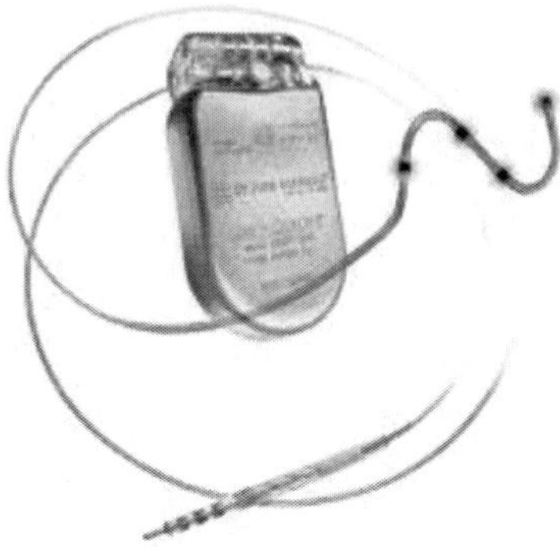

Figure 1. The St. Jude Quartet 1458Q quadripolar LV lead. Quartet is a trademark of St. Jude Medical, Inc. or its related companies. Reprinted with permission of St. Jude MedicalTM, © 2012. All rights reserved.

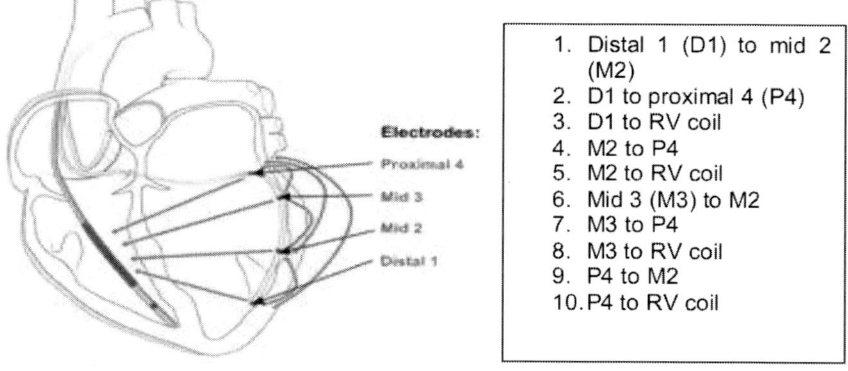

Figure 2. Ten vector configurations are available. Quartet is a trademark of St. Jude Medical, Inc. or its related companies. Reprinted with permission of St. Jude MedicalTM, © 2012. All rights reserved.

Mapping or Scar Imaging

As seen in the previous chapter, one of the predictors of non-response to CRT was underlying ischaemic heart disease, particularly the amount of scar burden in the posterolateral region [30, 31]. Scar in this region limits optimal positioning of the LV lead, causing high thresholds, and inadequate resynchronization [31]. We have already seen that various imaging techniques can be used to effectively map the left ventricular myocardium beforehand. This could help assess the amount of scar, regions of scar and transmurality of scar, allowing knowledge beforehand of optimal pacing sites to best improve resynchronization, and inform us of which areas to avoid. Certainly the new kid on the block in imaging with respect to this is cardiac magnetic resonance (CMR). Recent articles do suggest that prior imaging with CMR seems to predict clinical response and long term prognosis following CRT [32, 33]. Despite this the operator is still limited by coronary venous anatomy – even with prior imaging, the LV lead can only be placed down whichever branch is available.

Perhaps prior imaging with CMR could be used to predict which patients may be non-responders and in this group alternatives such as endocardial or multisite pacing could be considered. Certainly there needs to be better patient selection and criteria need to be refined and parameters that best define response and non-response clarified in order to address the issue of non-response. Other imaging modalities that have also shown promise in identifying scar and predicting CRT non-response include single photon emission CT myocardial perfusion imaging [34]. Further studies could help improve our understanding of non-response and provide better prediction criteria for the cardiologist in the future in appropriately selecting and assessing the patient for CRT.

Leadless Technology

Perhaps one of the most exciting advances of late is that of leadless pacemakers, which may help to dramatically change the face of pacing technology in the not too distant future. One of the main problems with all modern devices remains complications related to the pacing lead such as infection, fracture and dislodgement which necessitates further procedures such as lead repositioning, system revisions and extractions, a procedure with considerable risk to the patient. It therefore seems logical and highly desirable to develop a pacing system that eliminates the lead as the conduit for energy transfer.

Novel technology has therefore now been developed that uses ultrasound or magnetic field-mediated energy rather than the flow of electricity down a conductor in a pacing lead [35, 36]. A leadless pacing system includes an ultrasound generator implanted subcutaneously in the acoustic window of the chest wall and an endocardial receiver electrode, which is delivered to the target heart chamber and implanted into the endocardium directly using a steerable trans-vascular catheter. This uses the mechanical to electrical properties of piezoelectric materials for the transformation of acoustic to electrical energy to capture and pace the heart muscle. The safety and acute efficacy of this ultrasound mediated leadless technology has been valuated successfully in animal models for biventricular pacing [37].The efficacy and safety of the Wireless Cardiac Stimulation LV System (WiCS ®, EBR Systems, Inc., Sunnyvale, CA) are being evaluated in human implants in the ongoing WISE CRT trial [38].

For leadless CRT a further receiver electrode will have to be implanted in the LV endocardium following trans-septal puncture. A leadless pacing system has the advantages that it is less invasive, making implants potentially simpler, less time- consuming and technically less challenging, exposing the patient to less radiation, with fewer acute and chronic complications such as infection and skin erosion. It also has better patient aesthetics, and should allow lower cost and reduced length of hospital stay, and overcomes problems related to the lead such as fracture and dislodgement. Whilst the reliability of this technique to provide sustained energy over a prolonged period of time is currently unproven, other disadvantages include larger diameter catheters that are needed for implantation, It is also difficult to explant or reposition, and therefore must be abandoned at end of service. It also potentially has the adverse event of device dislodgement and embolisation, though theoretically it should become endothelialised after a certain period of time. All these will have to be taken account for and technology further developed and refined, but certainly leadless pacing systems appear a very real and attractive prospect for the future of pacing and CRT, and its arrival on the clinical scene is much anticipated.

Bio-Pacemakers

Following leadless systems, perhaps the next logical step would be to eliminate all pacing hardware altogether. This could potentially be done by bio-pacemaker generation. Whilst still very much in the research stages, the details of which are beyond the scope of this book, in principle bio-pacemaker generation can be achieved by either inducing pacemaker activity in normally quiescent ("working") myocardium or implanting exogenous cells engineered to sustain pacemaker activity ("cell based" approach), once electrically connected to the host myocardium [39]. This could theoretically be performed by injecting cells (perhaps stem cells, or gene therapy to deliver recombinant genes that activate specific ion channels or currents) via a catheter positioned from the femoral vein into the appropriate region of the heart (e.g the sinus node) to activate or stimulate the patient's own conduction system. Whilst still perhaps just a researcher's dream, this may provide a vision of the future to come, where medical technology advances to a point where we can simply restore normal physiology, where treatment is simple and effective, with little in the way of side effects and complications.

Whilst it remains to be seen if most of these novel ideas and developments will fully blossom from their embryonic stages to see the full light of day in our lifetimes, but certainly these are exciting times in the story of cardiac resynchronisation therapy.

REFERENCES

[1] Auricchio A, Prinzen FW. Non-responders to cardiac resynchronization therapy: the magnitude of the problem and the issues. *Circ. J.* 2011;75(3):521-7.

[2] Zaca V, Mondillo S, Gaddi R, et al. Profiling cardiac resynchronization therapy patients: responders, non-responders and those who cannot respond--the good, the bad and the ugly? *Int. J. Cardiovasc. Imaging* 2011 Jan;27(1):51-7.

[3] Daubert JC, Saxon L, Adamson PB, et al. 2012 EHRA/HRS expert consensus statement on cardiac resynchronization therapy in heart failure: implant and follow-up recommendations and management. *Heart Rhythm* 2012 Sep; 9(9):1524-76.

[4] del GM, Marini M, Bonmassari R. Implantation of a biventricular implantable cardioverter-defibrillator guided by an electroanatomic mapping system. *Europace* 2012 Jan;14(1):107-11.

[5] Rivero-Ayerza M, Van BY, Mekel J, et al. Left ventricular lead implantation assisted by magnetic navigation in a patient with a persistent left superior vena cava. *Int. J. Cardiol.* 2007 Mar 2;116(1):e15-e17.

[6] Rivero-Ayerza M, Thornton AS, Theuns DA, et al. Left ventricular lead placement within a coronary sinus side branch using remote magnetic navigation of a guidewire: a feasibility study. *J. Cardiovasc. Electrophysiol.* 2006 Feb;17(2):128-33.

[7] Rivero-Ayerza M, Jessurun E, Ramcharitar S, et al. Magnetically guided left ventricular lead implantation based on a virtual three-dimensional reconstructed image of the coronary sinus. *Europace* 2008 Sep;10(9):1042-7.

[8] Gallagher P, Martin L, Angel L, et al. Initial clinical experience with cardiac resynchronization therapy utilizing a magnetic navigation system. *J. Cardiovasc. Electrophysiol.* 2007 Feb;18(2):174-80.

[9] Lau EW. Achieving permanent left ventricular pacing-options and choice. *Pacing Clin. Electrophysiol.* 2009 Nov;32(11):1466-77.

[10] Mischke K, Knackstedt C. *Cardiac Resynchronization Therapy: Lead Positioning and Technical Advances*. In: Min M, editor. *Cardiac Pacemakers - Biological Aspects, Clinical Applications and Possible Complications*. InTech, 2011. p. 97-112.

[11] van DC, van G, I, Rademakers LM, et al. Left ventricular endocardial pacing improves resynchronization therapy in canine left bundle-branch hearts. *Circ. Arrhythm Electrophysiol.* 2009 Oct;2(5):580-7.

[12] Spragg DD, Dong J, Fetics BJ, et al. Optimal left ventricular endocardial pacing sites for cardiac resynchronization therapy in patients with ischemic cardiomyopathy. *J. Am. Coll. Cardiol.* 2010 Aug 31;56 (10):774-81.

[13] Derval N, Steendijk P, Gula LJ, et al. Optimizing hemodynamics in heart failure patients by systematic screening of left ventricular pacing sites: the lateral left ventricular wall and the coronary sinus are rarely the best sites. *J. Am. Coll. Cardiol.* 2010 Feb 9;55(6):566-75.

[14] Bracke FA, Houthuizen P, Rahel BM, et al. Left ventricular endocardial pacing improves the clinical efficacy in a non-responder to cardiac resynchronization therapy: role of acute haemodynamic testing. *Europace* 2010 Jul;12(7):1032-4.

[15] Bordachar P, Derval N, Ploux S, et al. Left ventricular endocardial stimulation for severe heart failure. *J. Am. Coll. Cardiol.* 2010 Aug 31;56(10):747-53.

[16] Bracke FA, van Gelder BM, Dekker LR, et al. Left ventricular endocardial pacing in cardiac resynchronisation therapy: Moving from bench to bedside. *Neth Heart J.* 2012 Mar;20(3):118-24.

[17] van Gelder BM, Houthuizen P, Scheffer MG, et al. Left Ventricular Endocardial Pacing Techniques as an Alternative for Ineffective Cardiac Resynchronization Therapy and the Role of Acute Hemodynamic Evaluation. In: Das MK, editor. *Modern Pacemakers - Present and Future*. InTech, 2011.

[18] Kassai I, Foldesi C, Szekely A, et al. New method for cardiac resynchronization therapy: transapical endocardial lead implantation for left ventricular free wall pacing. *Europace* 2008 Jul;10(7):882-3.
[19] Auricchio A, Prinzen FW. Cardiac resynchronization therapy: the more pacing sites, the better the outcome? *J. Am. Coll. Cardiol.* 2008 Apr 15;51(15):1463-5.
[20] Yoshida K, Yokoyama Y, Seo Y, et al. Triangle ventricular pacing in a non-responder to conventional bi-ventricular pacing. *Europace* 2008 Apr;10(4):502-4.
[21] Hof MJ, Maass AH. Leads for cardiac resynchronization therapy: where and how many? *Eur. J. Heart Fail* 2012 May;14(5):459-60.
[22] Leclercq C, Gadler F, Kranig W, et al. A randomized comparison of triple-site versus dual-site ventricular stimulation in patients with congestive heart failure. *J. Am. Coll. Cardiol.* 2008 Apr 15;51(15):1455-62.
[23] Cazeau S, Ritter P, Bakdach S, et al. Four chamber pacing in dilated cardiomyopathy. *Pacing Clin. Electrophysiol.* 1994 Nov;17(11 Pt 2):1974-9.
[24] Singh JP, Gras D. Biventricular pacing: current trends and future strategies. *Eur Heart J* 2012 Feb;33(3):305-13.
[25] Kamath GS, Balaram S, Choi A, et al. Long-term outcome of leads and patients following robotic epicardial left ventricular lead placement for cardiac resynchronization therapy. *Pacing Clin. Electrophysiol.* 2011 Feb;34(2):235-40.
[26] Biffi M, Moschini C, Bertini M, et al. Phrenic stimulation: a challenge for cardiac resynchronization therapy. *Circ. Arrhythm Electrophysiol.* 2009 Aug;2(4):402-10.
[27] Shetty AK, Duckett SG, Bostock J, et al. Use of a quadripolar left ventricular lead to achieve successful implantation in patients with previous failed attempts at cardiac resynchronization therapy. *Europace* 2011 Jul;13(7):992-6.
[28] Burger H, Schwarz T, Ehrlich W, et al. New generation of transvenous left ventricular leads - first experience with implantation of multipolar left ventricular leads. *Exp. Clin. Cardiol.* 2011;16(1):23-6.
[29] Thibault B, Karst E, Ryu K, et al. Pacing electrode selection in a quadripolar left heart lead determines presence or absence of phrenic nerve stimulation. *Europace* 2010 May;12(5):751-3.

[30] Bleeker GB, Kaandorp TA, Lamb HJ, et al. Effect of posterolateral scar tissue on clinical and echocardiographic improvement after cardiac resynchronization therapy. *Circulation* 2006 Feb 21;113(7):969-76.

[31] Ypenburg C, Schalij MJ, Bleeker GB, et al. Impact of viability and scar tissue on response to cardiac resynchronization therapy in ischaemic heart failure patients. *Eur. Heart J.* 2007 Jan;28(1):33-41.

[32] Leyva F. Cardiac resynchronization therapy guided by cardiovascular magnetic resonance. *J. Cardiovasc. Magn. Reson.* 2010;12:64.

[33] Taylor AJ, Elsik M, Broughton A, et al. Combined dyssynchrony and scar imaging with cardiac magnetic resonance imaging predicts clinical response and long-term prognosis following cardiac resynchronization therapy. *Europace* 2010 May;12(5):708-13.

[34] Adelstein EC, Saba S. Scar burden by myocardial perfusion imaging predicts echocardiographic response to cardiac resynchronization therapy in ischemic cardiomyopathy. *Am. Heart J.* 2007 Jan;153(1):105-12.

[35] Lee KL, Lau CP, Tse HF, et al. First human demonstration of cardiac stimulation with transcutaneous ultrasound energy delivery: implications for wireless pacing with implantable devices. *J. Am. Coll. Cardiol.* 2007 Aug 28;50(9):877-83.

[36] Kapa S, Bruce CJ, Friedman PA, et al. Advances in cardiac pacing: beyond the transvenous right ventricular apical lead. *Cardiovasc. Ther.* 2010 Dec;28(6):369-79.

[37] Echt DS, Cowan MW, Riley RE, et al. Feasibility and safety of a novel technology for pacing without leads. *Heart Rhythm* 2006 Oct;3(10):1202-6.

[38] DeFaria YD, Lonergan KL, Fu D, et al. Clinical factors and echocardiographic techniques related to the presence, size, and location of acoustic windows for leadless cardiac pacing. *Europace* 2011 Dec;13(12):1760-5.

[39] De Bakker JMT, Zaza A. Special issue on biopacemaking: clinically attractive, scientifically a challenge. *Med. Bio. Eng. Comput.* 2007;45:115-8.

Chapter 8

Case Studies

Case 1

A 58 year old male was assessed in follow up CRT clinic. He has a background of previous myocardial infarction ten years prior which left him with severely impaired systolic function (EF < 30%). He also has a history of type II diabetes, hypercholesterolaemia, hypertension and is an ex-smoker.

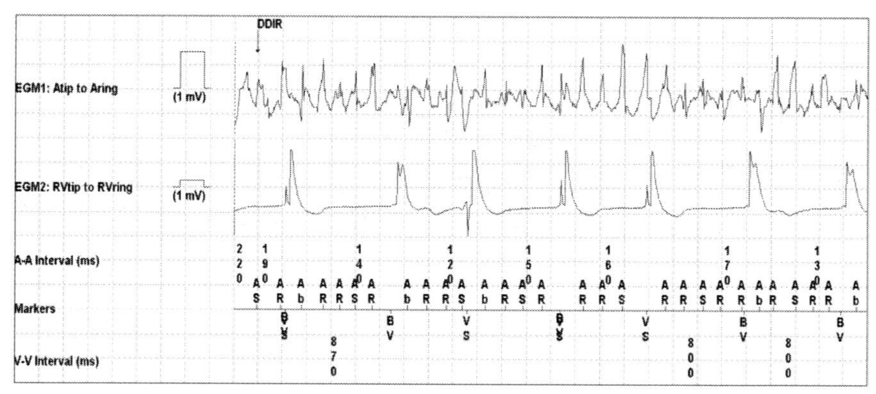

Pacing	% of Time since 29-Aug-2011.
AS-VS	20.7%
AS-VP	78.8%
AP-VS	< 0.1%
AP-VP	0.5%.

Figure 1.

He had primary prevention CRT-D implanted in 2005 due to NYHA class III symptoms (despite being on optimal medical therapy) and having a QRS duration of 155ms. His symptoms improved following the implant and he remained stable for some time. His device was checked through the pacing system analyser (PSA) in the clinic and electrograms can be seen in figure 1. On talking to the patient he admitted to worsening breathlessness over the last few months which the GP had been managing with diuretics.

Q1. What do the electrograms show?

Q2. What would be the appropriate management for this?

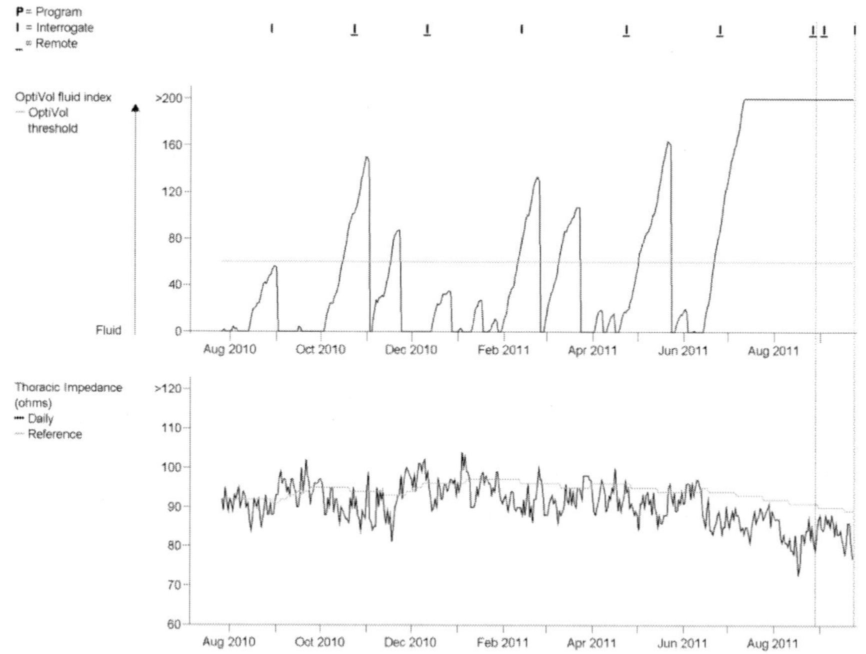

Case 1: Answer

The electrograms show that the patient is in atrial fibrillation (AF) with poorly controlled ventricular rate, and is subsequently BiV pacing less than 90%, the combination of which has led to a deterioration in his clinical condition, with worsening breathlessness. The OptiVol Fluid assessment also shows fluid accumulation as a result of decompensation of his heart failure.

AF is strongly associated with heart failure, occurring in about 50% of patients with NYHA class IV heart failure and is associated with increased morbidity and mortality [1].

Certainly the patient needs to be anti-coagulated with warfarin given the high thrombo-embolic risk with his heart failure. Diuretic doses will need to be increased or given intravenously to facilitate diuresis and off-loading of fluid to relieve pulmonary congestion. Increasing the amount of block at the AV node by increasing β-blockers and adding in digoxin may help control the ventricular rate and increase the % BiV pacing. In this case, the patient was already on optimum doses of medications. Simply increasing medications are also often ineffective in adequately controlling the rate and quickly stabilising the clinical condition. In such situations, if the atrial fibrillation is of recent onset, then performing DC cardioversion (once the patient is appropriately anti-coagulated) to electrically restore sinus rhythm may be of help. Often, though, given the advanced structural heart disease, attempts at cardioversion can be unsuccessful with the patient remaining in chronic atrial fibrillation. In such cases, performing AV node ablation will be suitable to help significantly increase BiV pacing to confer maximum benefit from CRT. There is an emerging body of literature to suggest that this approach should be considered more often in such patients as it confers significant clinical benefit [2-4].

References

[1] Maisel WH, Stevenson LW. Atrial fibrillation in heart failure: epidemiology, pathophysiology, and rationale for therapy. *Am. J. Cardiol.* 2003; 91 (6): 2-8.

[2] Gasparini M, Regoli F, Galimberti P, Ceriotti C, Cappelleri A. Cardiac resynchronization therapy in heart failure patients with atrial fibrillation. *Europace* 2009; 11: 82 – 86.

[3] Gasparini M, Auricchio A, Regoli F, Fantoni C, Kawabata M, Galimberti P, Pini D, Ceriotti C, Gronda E, Klersy C, Fratini S, Klein HH. Four year Efficacy of Cardiac Resynchronization Therapy on Exercise Tolerance and Disease Progression – The Importance of Performing Atrioventricular Junction Ablation in Patients with Atrial Fibrillation. *J. Am. Coll. Cardiol.* 2006; 48 (4): 734 – 743.

[4] Ganesan AN, Brooks AG, Roberts-Thomson KC, Lau DH, Kalman JM, Sandes P. Role of AV nodal ablation in cardiac resynchronization in

patients with coexistent atrial fibrillation and heart failure: a systematic review. *J. Am. Coll. Cardiol.* 2012; 59 (8): 719 – 726.

CASE 2

A 64 year old male with previous myocardial infarction, three vessel disease with severe left ventricular impairment with estimated EF of 25% with no viability, and LBBB on ECG underwent primary prevention biventricular ICD implantation as per NICE criteria. Procedure was uncomplicated, with Ability 4296 LV lead placed in suitable lateral branch. Pacing parameters and post procedure checks were satisfactory, and he was subsequently discharged the following day.

He returned shortly afterwards with intractable diaphragmatic twitch which would not settle fully despite altering pacemaker programming. A further procedure was performed to correct this and the post procedure chest X-ray can be seen below. His symptoms settled fully and following this he was discharged home. He has reported no further symptoms on follow up in pacing clinic.

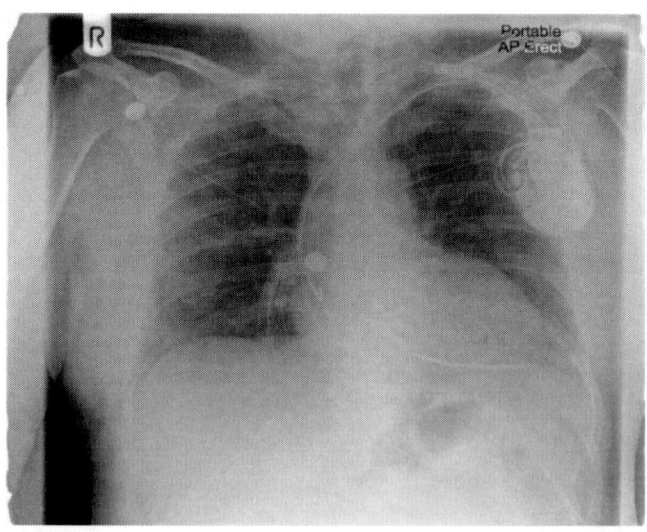

Questions: What procedure was performed? How was the twitch resolved?

Case 2: Answer

The old Ability 4296 lead has been removed from the lateral branch and a new St. Jude 1458Q Quartet lead inserted, this time in a postero-lateral branch, as can be seen on the chest X-ray. Diaphragmatic twitch is not uncommon, occurring in about 22% of patients with CRT implants [1], and is related to the proximity of the LV lead lying on the lateral wall of the left ventricle close to the left phrenic nerve. The St Jude Quartet model 1458Q, a quadripolar LV lead, can overcome these problems by allowing ten different pacing vectors (see figure 2) so the programmer can "electronically reposition" and change the electrode configuration to help avoid phrenic nerve stimulation and optimise pacing thresholds without having to adjust lead position manually [2-4]. In cases of resistant diaphragmatic twitching, certainly this LV lead can be considered and programming performed through an appropriate vector to resolve phrenic nerve stimulation and also allow satisfactory pacing parameters.

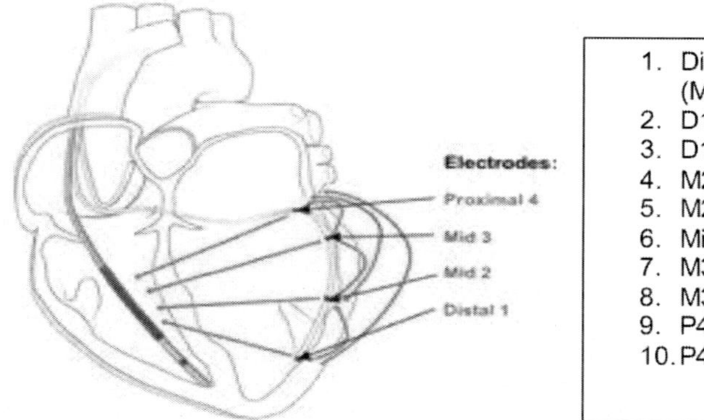

1. Distal 1 (D1) to mid 2 (M2)
2. D1 to proximal 4 (P4)
3. D1 to RV coil
4. M2 to P4
5. M2 to RV coil
6. Mid 3 (M3) to M2
7. M3 to P4
8. M3 to RV coil
9. P4 to M2
10. P4 to RV coil

Figure 2. The quadripolar LV lead allows ten pacing configurations to electronically programme a pacing vector that will allow satisfactory BiV pacing and avoid phrenic nerve stimulation / diaphragmatic twitching.

References

[1] Biffi M, Moschini C, Bertini M, Saporito D, Ziacchi M, DiembergerI, et al. Phrenic stimulation: a challenge for cardiac resynchronization therapy. *Circ. Arrhythm Electrophysiol.* 2009; 2: 402 – 410.

[2] Shetty AK, Duckett SG, Bostock J, Rosenthal E, Rinaldi CA. Use of a quadripolar left ventricular lead to achieve successful implantation in

patients with previous failed attempts at cardiac resynchronization therapy. *Europace* 2011; 13: 992 – 996.

[3] Burger H, Schwarz T, Ehrlich W, Sperzel J, Kloevekorn WP, Ziegelhoeffer T. New generation of transvenous left ventricular leads – first experience with implantation of multipolar left ventricular leads. *Exp. Clin. Cardiol.* 2011; 16(1): 23 – 26.

[4] Thibault B, Karst E, Ryu K, Paiement P, Farazi TG. Pacing electrode selection in a quadripolar left heart lead determines presence or absence of phrenic nerve stimulation. *Europace* 2010; 12(5): 751 – 753.

CASE 3

An 83 year old male with a background of hypertension, chronic atrial fibrillation, previous stroke, hypothyroidism and benign prostatic hypertrophy, had VVI pacemaker inserted few years back for slow AF with pauses causing dizziness. He was under regular follow up and subsequently went on to have an upgrade of device from VVI to bi-ventricular pacemaker due to unopposed RV pacing causing worsening of LV function and symptoms of breathlessness, which was performed last year.

Battery Voltage

(RRT=2.77V)
30-Sep-2011
Voltage 2.97 V

Remaining Longevity

Estimated at:	2.5 years
Minimum:	1.5 years
Maximum:	3.5 years

(based on initial interrogation)

Sensing Integrity Counter

(if >300 counts, check for sensing issues)
Since 26-Sep-2011
Short V-V Intervals 0

Lead Impedance

A. Pacing	(Unipolar)	>3000 ohms	16-Nov-2010
RV Pacing	(Bipolar)	532 ohms	30-Sep-2011
LV Pacing	(LVtip to Can)	513 ohms	30-Sep-2011

Sensing

P-Wave Amplitude	2.6 mV	30-Sep-2011
R-Wave Amplitude	8.0 mV	22-Aug-2011

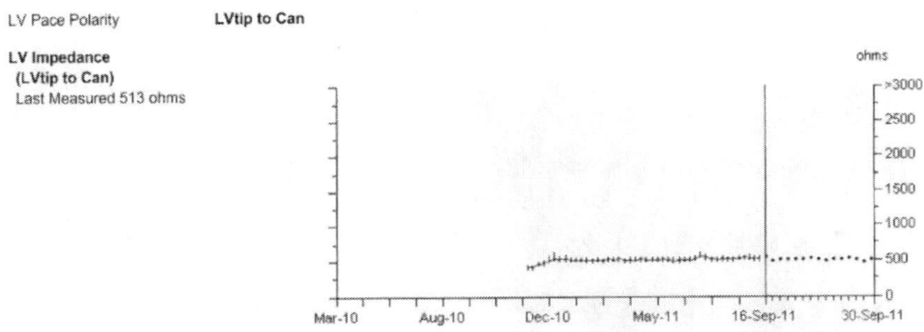

Figure 3.

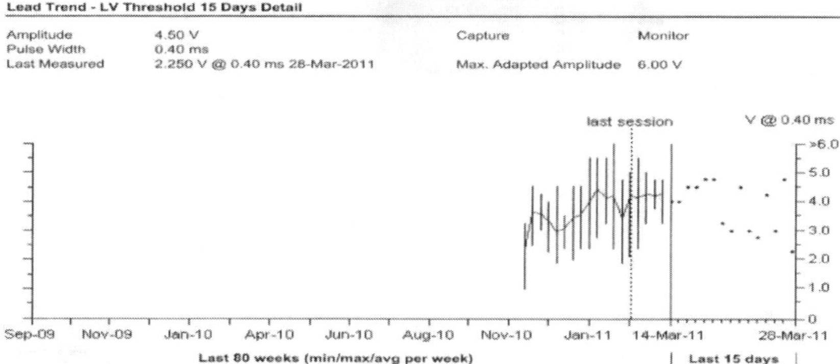

The procedure was uneventful with Medtronic Ability 4196 bipolar LV lead being placed in a large suitable lateral branch. This was connected to a Medtronic CRT-P device, and the atrial port plugged. Post procedure checks were satisfactory and patient was discharged the next day. On follow up in pacing clinic he was found to have the following unusual findings on pacemaker check (see figure 3).

Question:

What does the pacemaker check show?

How can the problem be explained and how can it be corrected?

Case 3: Answer:

On reviewing the pacing check the first point to note is that the right ventricular sensing and impedance is satisfactory. The RV threshold is not mentioned here so it can be assumed that it is satisfactory as it is not relevant to the question – this is a book on CRT and therefore most questions will relate to the LV lead! The atrial impedance is above 3000 ohms as the atrial port is plugged, with there being no atrial lead as the patient is in AF.

The main point to note is that the LV threshold is extremely fluctuant and variable whilst the impedance has been steady and unchanged within satisfactory limits, suggesting that there is no problem or issue here with either insulation break or conductor fracture. Rather this is due to solely to the contact of the LV lead tip within the lateral vein branch. This unusual finding can be seen when a small sized LV lead has been placed in a particularly large vessel allowing the lead to move around more freely within the vessel, allowing varying contact with the lateral LV epicardium and hence fluctuating thresholds. It is important to ensure that the appropriate sized LV lead is placed in the appropriate sized vessel, and to confirm that there is good lead position, placement and stability during the procedure to try reduce this from occurring. If despite all this, the above scenario results, the problem can be addressed by increasing the pulse width, which was done in this particular case (see figure 4), resulting in more stable, less fluctuating LV thresholds. The other alternative (if the problem still persists) is to reposition the LV lead into a different branch.

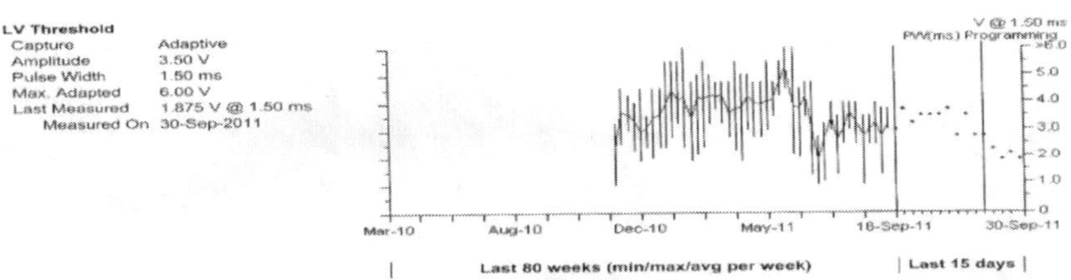

Figure 4. LV thresholds fluctuate less once pulse width increased to 1.50ms.

Case 4

A 65 year old male was transferred from a local district general hospital for insertion of a biventricular ICD. He had been admitted there following an out of hospital VF arrest and had been successfully resuscitated following bystander CPR and defibrillation from the paramedic crew with return of cardiac output.

Echocardiogram performed subsequently confirmed severe left ventricular systolic dysfunction, and coronary angiogram showed mild coronary artery disease but no flow limiting lesions. ECG showed sinus rhythm with T wave inversion in lateral leads.

Procedure was uncomplicated with Ability 4296 bipolar LV lead placed in good position in sizeable lateral vein. Pacing characteristics were excellent and DFT testing successful. He made good recovery and was discharged. He had been well for a while but later was seen in ICD clinic having had a shock from the device. Details from the device interrogation are shown (see figure 5 below).

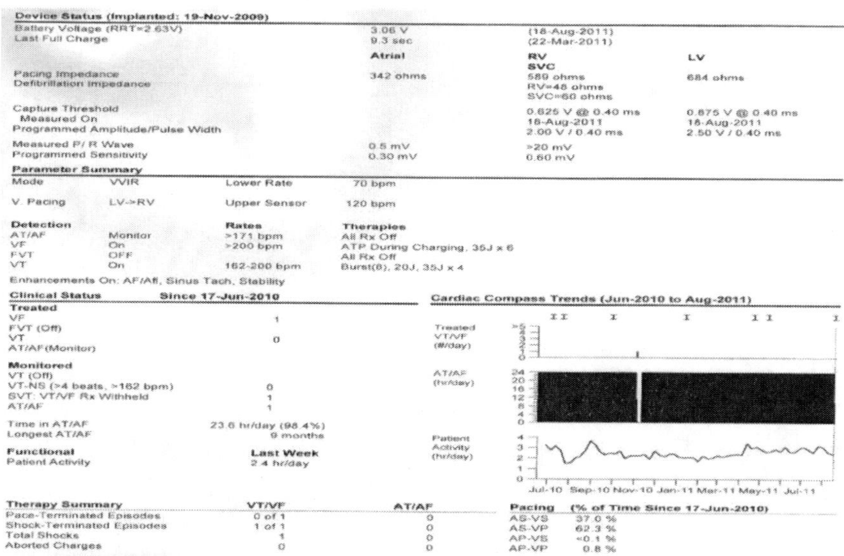

Device Status (Implanted: 19-Nov-2009)

Battery Voltage (RRT=2.63V)	3.06 V	(18-Aug-2011)	
Last Full Charge	9.3 sec	(22-Mar-2011)	
	Atrial	**RV** / **SVC**	**LV**
Pacing Impedance	342 ohms	589 ohms	684 ohms
Defibrillation Impedance		RV=48 ohms, SVC=60 ohms	
Capture Threshold		0.625 V @ 0.40 ms	0.875 V @ 0.40 ms
Measured On		18-Aug-2011	18-Aug-2011
Programmed Amplitude/Pulse Width		2.00 V / 0.40 ms	2.50 V / 0.40 ms
Measured P/ R Wave	0.5 mV	>20 mV	
Programmed Sensitivity	0.30 mV	0.60 mV	

Parameter Summary

Mode	VVIR	Lower Rate	70 bpm
V. Pacing	LV->RV	Upper Sensor	120 bpm

Detection		**Rates**	**Therapies**
AT/AF	Monitor	>171 bpm	All Rx Off
VF	On	>200 bpm	ATP During Charging, 35J x 6
FVT	OFF		All Rx Off
VT	On	162-200 bpm	Burst(8), 20J, 35J x 4

Enhancements On: AF/Afl, Sinus Tach, Stability

Clinical Status **Since 17-Jun-2010**

Treated	
VF	1
FVT (Off)	
VT	0
AT/AF(Monitor)	
Monitored	
VT (Off)	
VT-NS (>4 beats, >162 bpm)	0
SVT: VT/VF Rx Withheld	1
AT/AF	1
Time in AT/AF	23.6 hr/day (98.4%)
Longest AT/AF	9 months
Functional	**Last Week**
Patient Activity	2.4 hr/day

Cardiac Compass Trends (Jun-2010 to Aug-2011)

Therapy Summary	**VT/VF**	**AT/AF**
Pace-Terminated Episodes	0 of 1	0
Shock-Terminated Episodes	1 of 1	0
Total Shocks	1	0
Aborted Charges	0	0

Pacing	**(% of Time Since 17-Jun-2010)**
AS-VS	37.0 %
AS-VP	62.3 %
AP-VS	<0.1 %
AP-VP	0.8 %

Figure 5.

Question:

What does the device interrogation show?

What further management needs to be done?

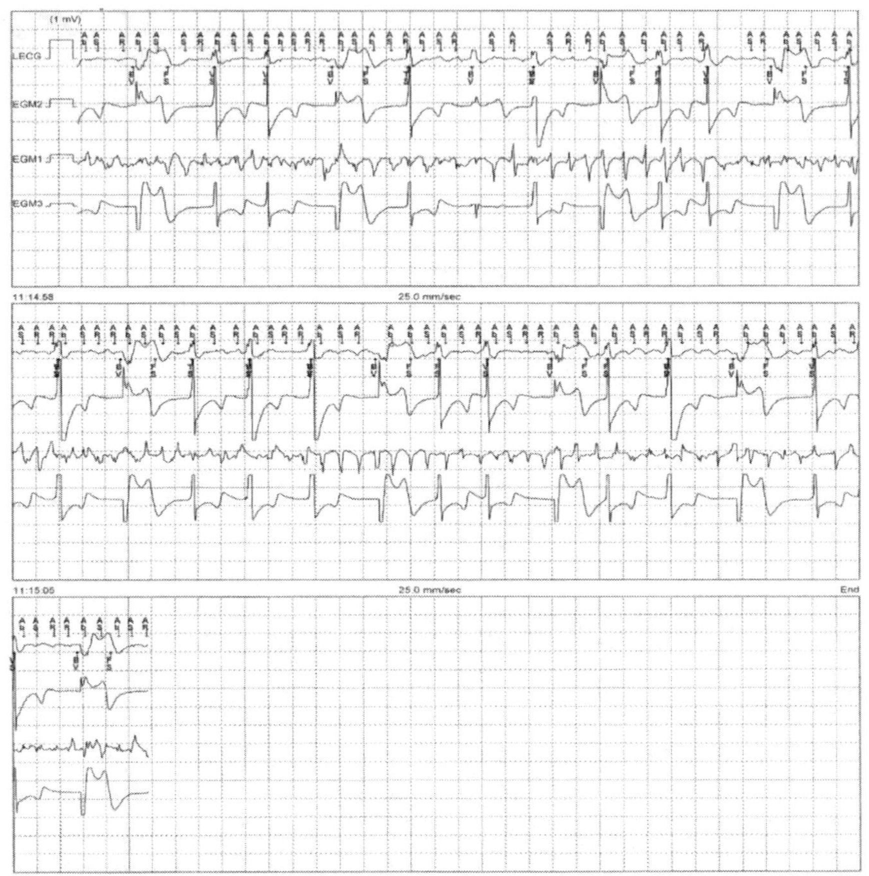

Case 4: Answer

The first point to note is that the patient is now in AF, as can be seen on the atrial electrogram, which mentioned as before, is very common in patients with advance heart failure. As a result he is BiV pacing much less than 90%. Again medications (e.g. b-blockers, digoxin) will need to be increased to cause more block at the AV node to improve % BiV pacing. Further treatment with DC cardioversion or referring for AV node ablation will need to be considered.

The pacing characteristics (impedances, thresholds etc) of the leads themselves are satisfactory. The other main finding here is that there is T wave over-sensing and in combination with his atrial fibrillation, lead to an inappropriate shock from the device.

Up to 15% of patients implanted with ICDs experience inappropriate shocks during the first year [1]. In 20%, the shocks are due to inadequate device sensing [2] and T wave sensing is the most common cause of ventricular over-sensing in 14% of cases [3]. Reversible causes of T wave abnormalities such as electrolyte disturbances, drugs and myocardial ischaemia needs to be excluded. Device reprogramming can be tried. If the intrinsic R-wave is very large and T-wave amplitude small, decreasing sensitivity to just greater than the T wave may solve the problem. Alternatively it may be possible to programme the auto-gain / adjust the slope of decay, or extend post pacing ventricular blanking periods to avoid T wave over-sensing.

In most cases, it is necessary to re-position the implanted lead, insert an additional lead for sensing, or implant a new generator [4]. The newer devices incorporate more advanced technology, (e.g. Medtronic SmartShock™ and St Jude Medical ShockGuard™) which uses more sophisticated algorithms to minimise T wave over-sensing and inappropriate device therapy as much as possible.

References

[1] Sweeney MO, Wathen MS, Volosin K, Abdalla I, DeGroot PJ, Otterness MF, Stark AJ. Appropriate and inappropriate ventricular therapies, quality of life, and mortality among primary and secondary prevention implantable cardioverter defibrillator patients: results from the Pacing Fast VT REduces Shock ThErapies (PainFREE Rx II) trial. *Circulation* 2005; 111 (22): 2898 -905.

[2] Daubert JP, Zareba W, Cannom DS, McNitt S, Rosero SZ, Wang P, Schuger C, Steinberg JS, Higgins SL, Wilber DJ, Klein H, Andrews ML, Hall WJ, Moss AJ; MADIT II Investigators. *J. Am. Coll. Cardiol.* 2008; 51(14): 1357-65.

[3] Weretka S, Michaelsen J, Becker R, Karle CA, Voss F, Hilbel T, Osswald BR, Bahner ML, Senges JC, Kuebler W, Schoels W. Ventricular oversensing: a study of 101 patients implanted with dual chamber defibrillators and two different lead systems. *Pacing Clin. Electrophysiol* 2003; 26(1 Pt 1): 65-70.

[4] Frutos M, Pedrote A, Arana E, Sanchez-Brotons J. T-wave Oversensing with Inappropriate Therapy in Remote Monitoring. *Indian Pacing Electrophysiol. J.* 2010; 10(6): 274-277.

CASE 5

A 66 year old male with a background of ischaemic heart disease, chronic obstructive pulmonary disease (COPD), AF, LBBB, and previous ICD in situ was admitted with decompensated heart failure and worsening of his LV function. ICD check was satisfactory with no evidence of ventricular arrhythmias or shocks. Once medically stabilised, a decision was made to upgrade his device to a biventricular ICD and implant a LV lead given worsening of his heart failure. Procedure was uncomplicated with Medtronic 4296 LV lead placed in lateral branch of coronary sinus. There was some diaphragmatic twitching and poor capture when pacing in the bi-polar configuration but satisfactory parameters were obtained when pacing from the LV tip and the ring to the RV coil. A new CRT-D generator was implanted and patient discharged the next day. He remained well for a few weeks but was admitted feeling unwell shortly after. Further device interrogation is shown below (see figure 6).

Question:

What does the device interrogation show?

What could have caused this? What could be done to check if this is the case?

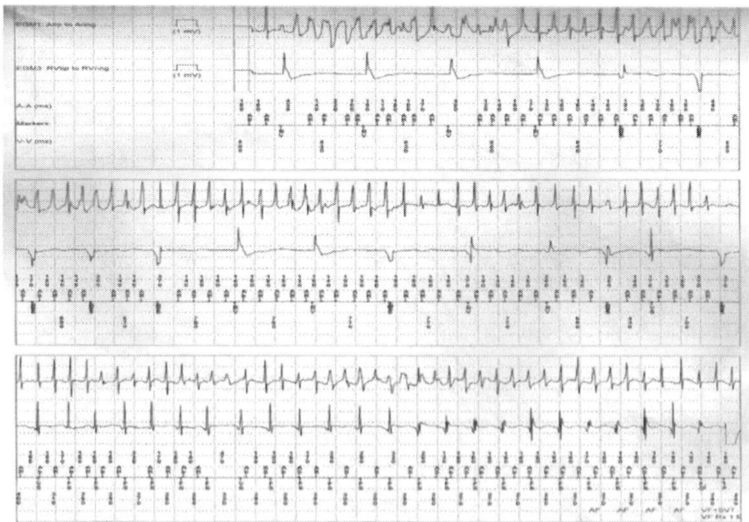

Figure 6.

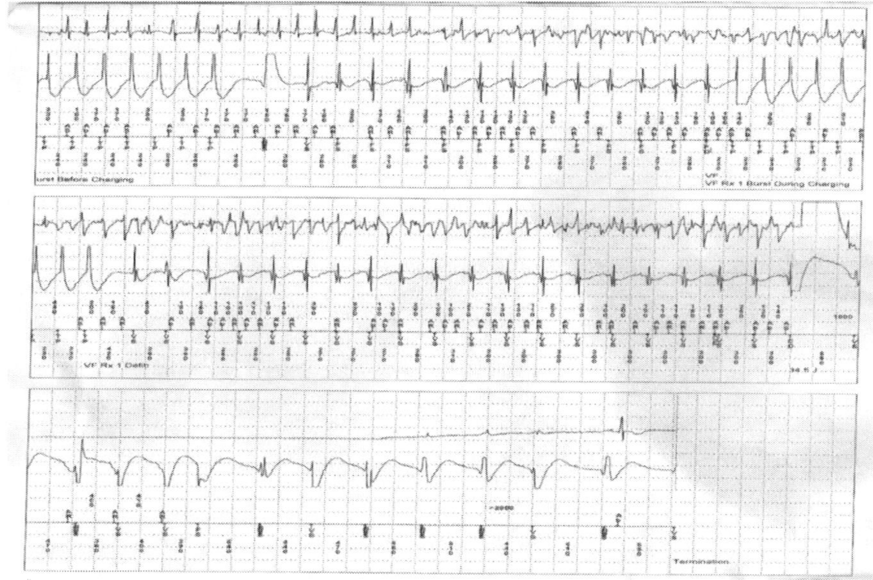

Case 5: Answer

The atrial electrogram shows that the patient is in established AF, as known previously from the history. The RV electrogram starts with BiV pacing but towards the bottom of the first strip patient goes into ventricular tachycardia (note the sudden increase in heart rate).

The device recognizes this and tries two runs of anti-tachycardia pacing (ATP). When this fails to terminate the ventricular tachycardia (VT), it delivers an appropriate shock. This terminates the VT as well as cardioverting the AF to sinus rhythm.

It is unusual that prior to the recent procedure the patient had had no therapies, but following the recent upgrade to biventricular ICD with insertion of a new LV lead he has subsequently developed VT, requiring device therapy. It is very possible that the LV pacing could be the cause of this – perhaps pacing around a region of scar could have triggered the VT. Certainly there were no abnormal investigation results to suggest otherwise.

Blood tests were normal, and CXR showed no lead displacement and pacing characteristics of all the leads was satisfactory on the device check. Interestingly once the LV lead was turned off, patient did not have any further episodes of VT. Repositioning of the LV lead is currently being considered.

CASE 6

An 83 year old female with a history of ischaemic cardiomyopathy, with severely impaired LV function, COPD, type II diabetes, and with biventricular ICD already in situ, attended for CRT-D generator change as battery was reaching ERI.

This was performed in October 2011. Procedure was uncomplicated and patient discharged home. In early to mid December 2011 she was asked to attend pacing clinic as Carelink download revealed a significant abnormality and triggered the alarm.

See figure 6. A chest X-ray was also performed and can be seen below.

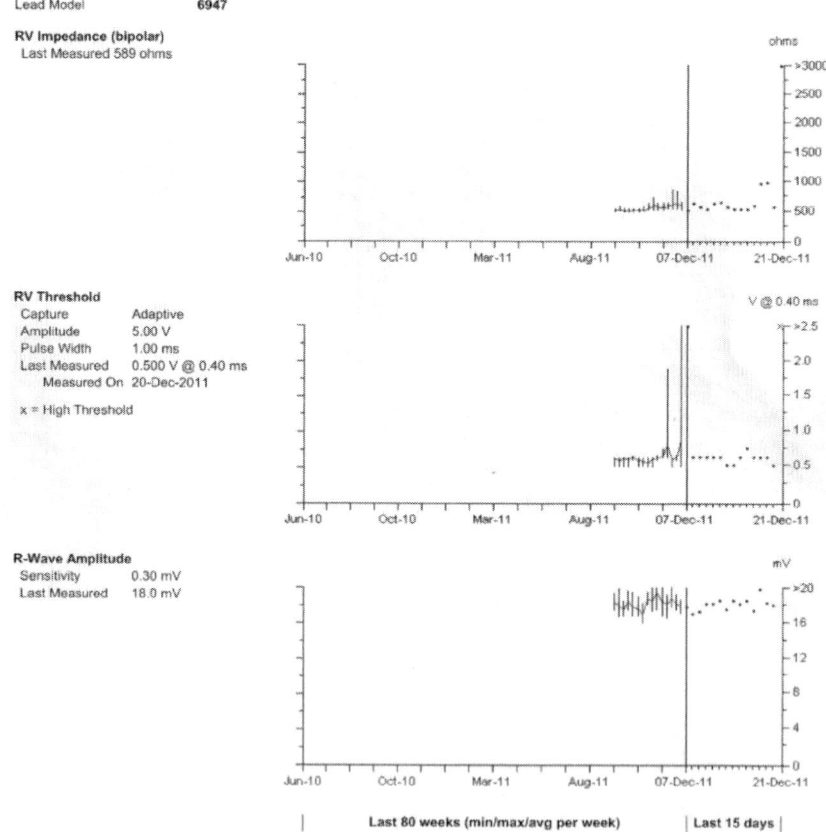

Figure 6.

Question:
What was the abnormality that caused the device to alarm?

What should be done next?

CASE 6

CXR Shown Below of Patient with Alarming Device

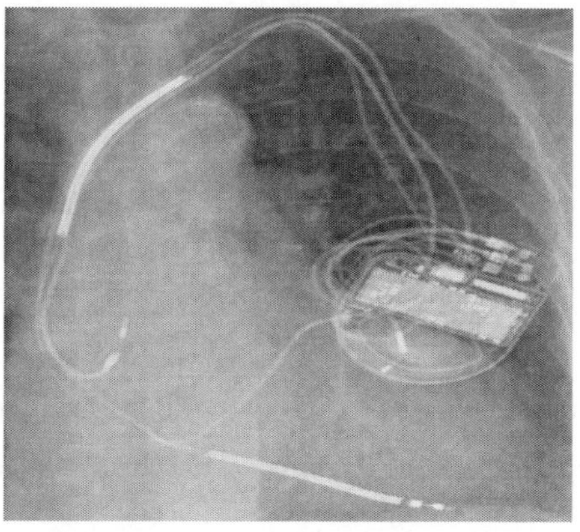

Case 6: Answer

The device check shows a sudden increase in RV lead impedance to > 3000 ohms on 19th Dec 2011 (last dot on the first lead impedance graph). This is why the device was alarming. The CXR shows no evidence of conductor fracture but on close examination it can be seen that the RV pin (the middle one in the CRT-D generator header) is not fully through the set screw. This is the cause of the very high RV lead impedance (the other main cause than can lead to high impedance is lead fracture). The patient was admitted urgently for reassessment and revision of the device with re-insertion of the RV lead pin properly into the device header to ensure good connection. Lead check was satisfactory. This promptly resolved the issue and the patient was sent home the day after. Further follow up in pacing clinics have been satisfactory with no further problems encountered. It is very important to ensure that when performing CRT-D box changes that all lead pins are advanced all the way through into their respective ports in the header before the set screw is tightened, and ensuring that there is a good, tight connection by visually assessing the device at the time of procedure or gently tugging at the leads to ensure that they are secured properly in the header. This helps to avoid a simple yet important and avoidable complication.

CASE 7

A 55 year old male was admitted with out of hospital cardiac arrest. He was shocked for ventricular fibrillation and successfully resuscitated. A subsequent echocardiogram showed severely impaired LV systolic function with ejection fraction less than 35%, and coronary angiogram revealed only minor coronary artery disease with no evidence of flow limiting lesions. ECG showed sinus rhythm with LBBB with QRS duration of 160ms. A decision was made to implant a CRT-D device. The procedure was uncomplicated and patient discharged not long after. He was seen in pacing clinic six weeks later, at which time he stated that he now felt his breathing had got significantly worse and was frustrated that the device was not working properly. Pacing check was satisfactory. Cine image of the recent procedure was reviewed (see figure 7 below).

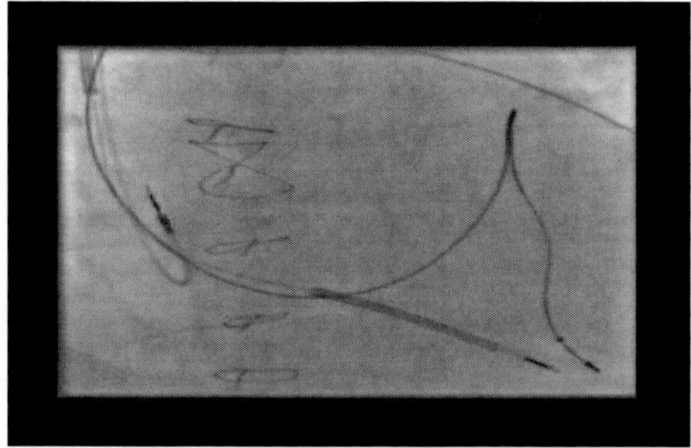

Figure 7.

Question:

What is the cause of non-response in this patient? How can it be corrected?

Case 7: Answer

About 20 - 30% of patients fail to respond to CRT [1], and this aspect of the procedure should be discussed with the patient in detail beforehand. Some patients may not notice a particular difference in their symptoms whilst some experience a worsening of symptoms. It is important to have a methodical, rigorous approach to assessing and managing the non-responder to look for any reversible causes. LV lead positioning, such as in this case, is a particularly important example [2, 3]. The LV lead should be positioned in a suitable lateral branch of the coronary sinus, so that the most delayed region of the LV myocardium is activated when re-synchronising the right and left ventricle, to confer the maximum clinical benefit. In this case, the LV lead has been positioned down an anterior vein, and it can be seen that there is not much distance at all (a desirable factor) between the RV and LV lead here to allow effective resynchronisation therapy. The patient attended for repeat procedure where the LV lead was re-positioned down a lateral branch (which was difficult but achievable) with good spacing between the RV and LV lead tips. See figure 8 below for the post procedure cine image, showing much better final position of the LV lead. Following this the patient noticed marked improvement in his symptoms. This case highlights the importance of the operator needing to be extremely meticulous and persistent in order to place the LV lead in the best possible position in the CRT patient to get the best outcome. Failure to do this (as in this case) can result in non-response and the need for a further procedure to reposition the lead.

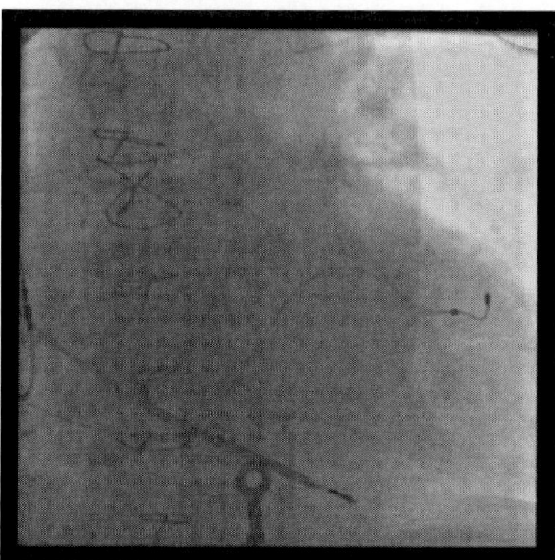

Figure 8. Post LV lead repositioning into a lateral branch.

References

[1] Auricchio A, Printzen FW. Non-Responders to Cardiac Resynchronisation Therapy – The Magnitude of the Problem and the Issues. *Circulation Journal* 2011; 75: 521 – 527.

[2] Gorcsan III, J. Finding Pieces of the Puzzle of Nonresponse to Cardiac Resynchronisation Therapy. *Circulation* 2011; 123: 10-12.

[3] Herre J. Keys to successful cardiac resynchronisation therapy. *Am. Heart J.* 2007; 153 (4): 518 – 524.

Case 8

A 62 year old male with ischaemic cardiomyopathy and severely impaired left ventricular systolic function, and NYHA class III heart failure despite optimum medical treatment, and LBBB, attended for CRT implantation. The procedure was very difficult. See images below.

Question: Why was the procedure so difficult? How was this overcome?

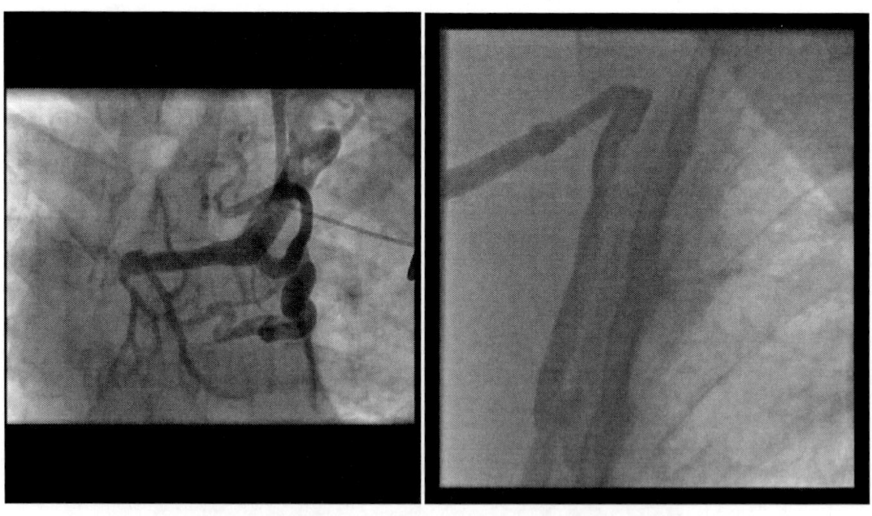

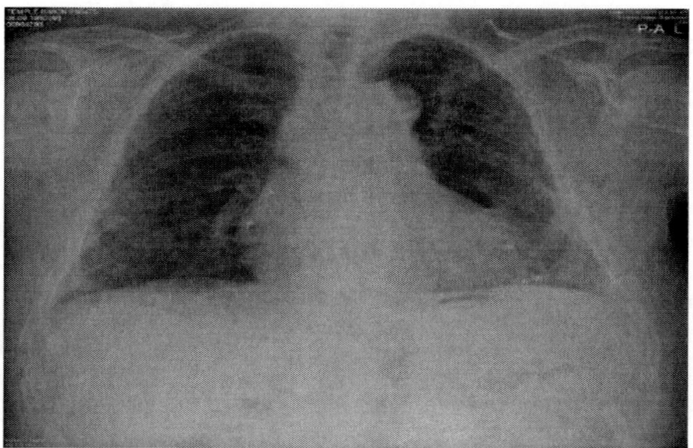

Case 8: Answer

The pictures above show venograms of both the left and right side in this patient.

These show anomalous venous drainage, with no superior vena cava and direct route to place transvenous pacing leads in the right ventricle and right atrium, let alone an LV lead into the coronary sinus. This makes it impossible to implant a CRT device by the traditional method, due to access to the heart limited by abnormal venous anatomy.

It is important to be aware that in approximately 5 out of every 100 CRT cases it may not be possible to place an LV lead due to variations in venous anatomy and poor or no suitable distal targets.

Whilst this case is unusual in that there is not even a straight forward route into the heart, it helps highlight that appropriate access can be a problem encountered in some cases. In this situation the patient was referred for a full epicardial CRT system which was implanted surgically, as can be seen in the chest X-ray below.

If the LV lead cannot be implanted through the coronary sinus, then the option of referral for surgical epicardial LV lead placement should always be considered.

CASE 9

A 72 year old male with ischaemic cardiomyopathy and severe LV systolic dysfunction had CRT-P device inserted. Procedure was uncomplicated, though the LV lead had been difficult to position. The initial selected branch did not give satisfactory parameters, and it had to be placed in a different lateral branch.

LV threshold here was still on the higher side but acceptable with programming a different pacing configuration. Post procedure chest X-ray and pacing checks are shown below.

Question: What is the main abnormal finding here?

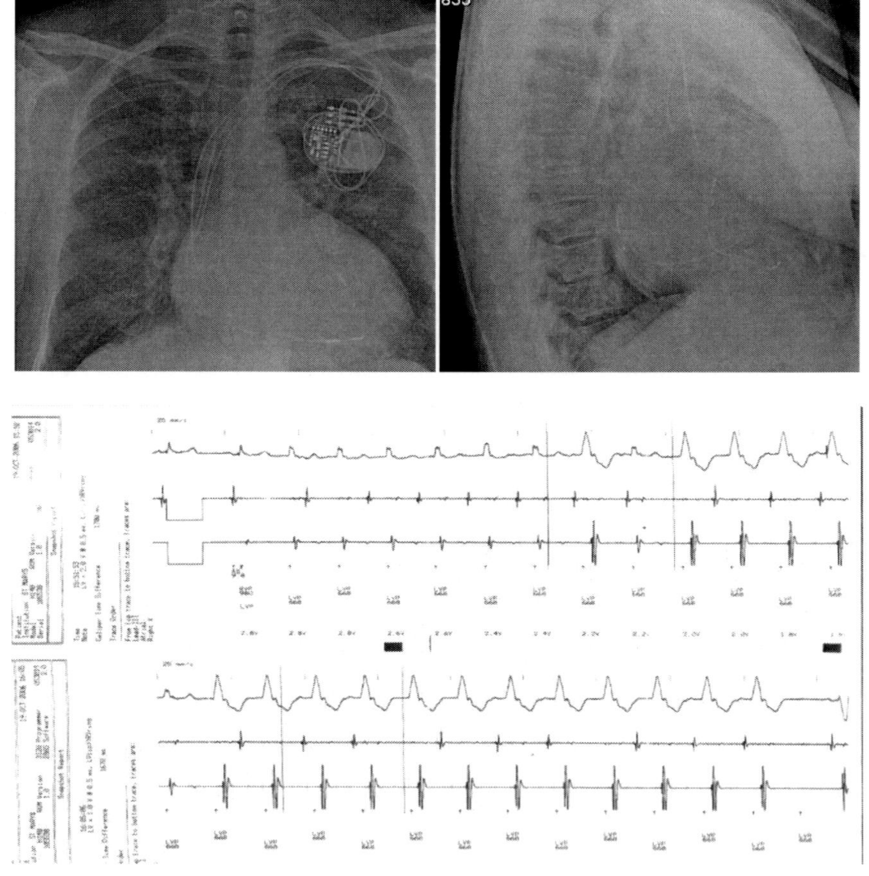

Case 9: Answer

The electrogram (EGM) demonstrates anodal capture. The chest X-rays confirm position of the LV lead. The device check shows surface ECG (top trace – lead III), atrial EGM (middle trace) and RV EGM (bottom trace), and that the LV pacing marker is associated with QRS morphology change consistent with RV or anodal capture. Standard bipolar pacing is between two closely spaced electrodes, such as LV lead tip to LV ring. Capture typically occurs at the cathode.

Modern CRT devices allow the option of programming LV lead pacing as LV tip electrode (cathode) to RV lead coil or ring (anode) as an alternative to improve pacing thresholds. Anodal stimulation is defined as capture at the pacing anode instead of cathode (i.e. the right ventricle). This is more common at higher pacing outputs. If anodal stimulation occurs when a CRT device is programmed LV tip to RV coil / ring, the RV is unintentionally captured instead of the LV. If not identified and corrected at the time of CRT implant, effective cardiac resynchronization will not occur and this may be a cause of non-response [1-3].

To avoid or correct anodal capture one should use a bipolar LV lead, use a pacing vector that avoids the RV ring (unipolar LV to RV coil or to can), or adjust the pacing output high enough to capture the LV but low enough not to capture the anodal RV [4].

REFERENCES

[1] Dendy KF, Powell BD, Cha YM, Espinosa RE, Friedman PA, Rea RF, Hayes DL, Redfield MM, Asirvatham SJ. Anodal Stimulation: An Underrecognized Cause of Nonresponders to Cardiac Resynchronization Therapy. *Indian Pacing and Electrophysiology Journal* 2011; 11(3): 64 – 72.

[2] Tamborero D, Mont L, Alanis R, et al. Anodal capture in cardiac resynchronization therapy implications for device programming. *Pacing Clin. Electrophysiol.* 2006; 29: 940 – 945.

[3] Thibault B, Roy D, Guerra PG, et al. Anodal right ventricular capture during left ventricular stimulation in CRT-implantable cardioverter defibrillators. *Pacing Clin. Electrophysiol.* 2005; 28: 613 – 619.

[4] Kashiwase K, Kobayashi H, Wada M, Nakanishi H, Hirata A, Ueda Y. Anodal Capture May Prevent Cardiac Resynchronization Therapy from Working Effectively. A Case Report of Left Ventricular Lead Dislodgement. *J. Arrhythmia* 2011; 27: 150 -153.

CASE 10

A 62 year old patient with CRT-D was followed up in pacemaker clinic. The device check was abnormal and subsequently a chest X-ray was performed. Both can be seen below.

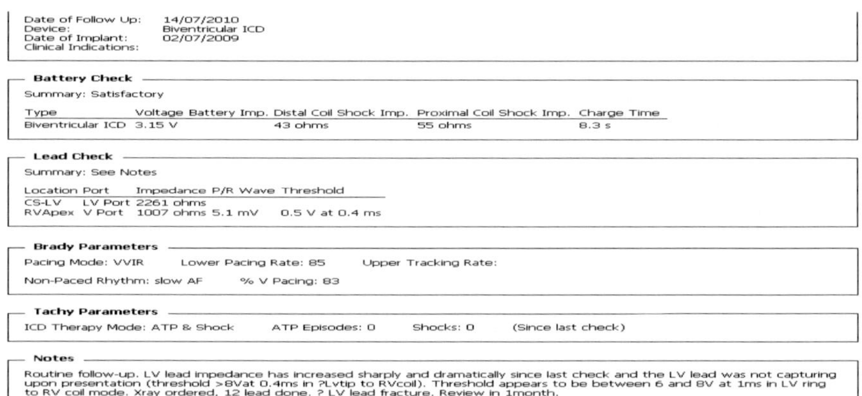

Date of Follow Up: 14/07/2010
Device: Biventricular ICD
Date of Implant: 02/07/2009
Clinical Indications:

Battery Check

Summary: Satisfactory

Type	Voltage	Battery Imp.	Distal Coil Shock Imp.	Proximal Coil Shock Imp.	Charge Time
Biventricular ICD	3.15 V		43 ohms	55 ohms	8.3 s

Lead Check

Summary: See Notes

Location	Port	Impedance	P/R Wave	Threshold
CS-LV	LV Port	2261 ohms		
RVApex	V Port	1007 ohms	5.1 mV	0.5 V at 0.4 ms

Brady Parameters

Pacing Mode: VVIR Lower Pacing Rate: 85 Upper Tracking Rate:

Non-Paced Rhythm: slow AF % V Pacing: 83

Tachy Parameters

ICD Therapy Mode: ATP & Shock ATP Episodes: 0 Shocks: 0 (Since last check)

Notes

Routine follow-up. LV lead impedance has increased sharply and dramatically since last check and the LV lead was not capturing upon presentation (threshold >8Vat 0.4ms in ?Lvtip to RVcoil). Threshold appears to be between 6 and 8V at 1ms in LV ring to RV coil mode. Xray ordered, 12 lead done. ? LV lead fracture. Review in 1month.

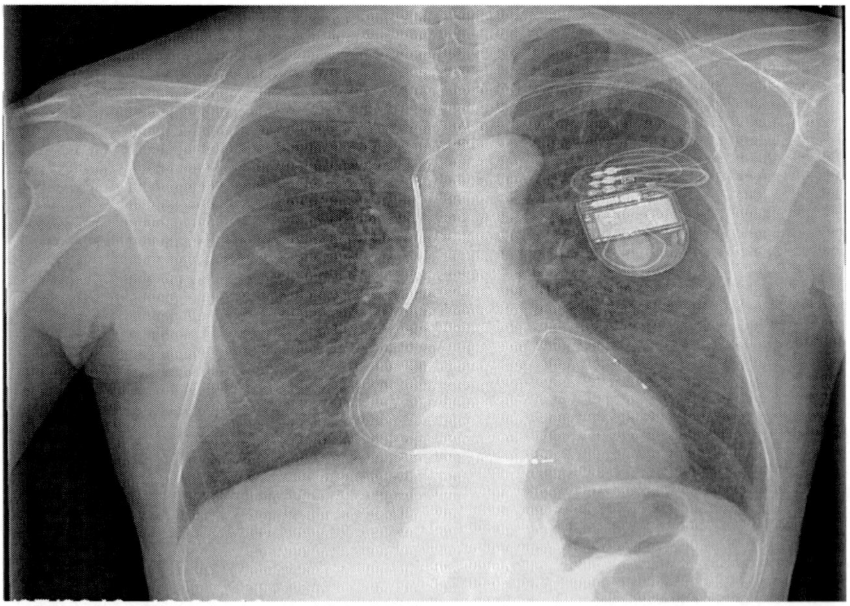

Question: What is the problem? What needs to be done?

Case 10: Answer

The device check shows that the LV lead impedance has increased sharply and is significantly raised (>2000 Ohms), and is also not capturing properly with thresholds being very high between 6 and 8V at 1ms. In this situation a chest X-ray needs to be performed and analysed carefully, particularly focussing on the lead looking for fracture.

If examined closely the chest X-ray here does indeed show fracture of the LV lead (seen on the right hand side of the picture just as the lead comes out of the device header).

The fractured LV lead will need to be removed and a new LV lead inserted in order for effective CRT to be restored, which was done in this case.

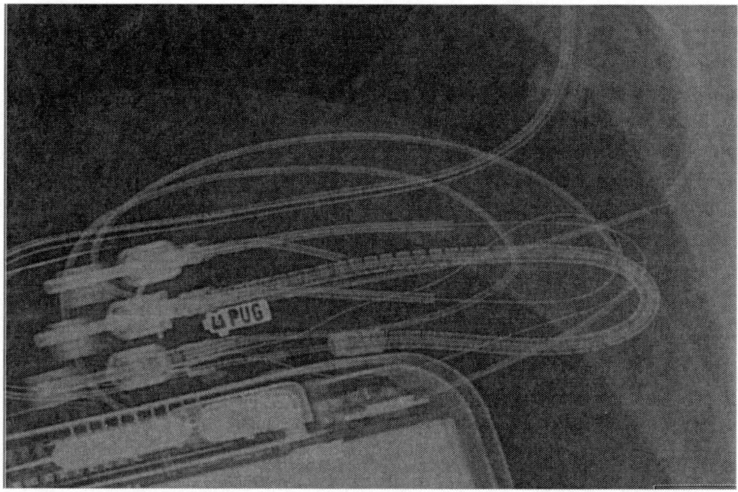

Figure 9. X-ray showing LV lead fracture.

INDEX

B

C

N

O

P

Q

R

S

T

U

V